The Recovery Philosophy and Direct Social Work Practice

Also available from Lyceum Books, Inc.

Advisory Editor: Thomas M. Meenaghan, *New York University*

Psychoeducation in Mental Health
by Joseph Walsh

Endings in Clinical Practice: Effective Closure in Diverse Settings,
Second edition
by Joseph Walsh

Understanding and Managing the Therapeutic Relationship
by Fred R. McKenzie

The Costs of Courage: Combat Stress, Warriors, and Family Survival
by Josephine G. Price, Col. David H. Price, and Kimberly K. Shackleford

Social Work with HIV and AIDS: A Practice-Based Guide
by Diana Rowan and Contributors

Lesbian and Gay Couples: Lives, Issues, and Practice
by Ski Hunter

Citizenship Social Work with Older People
by Malcolm Payne

Character Formation and Identity in Adolescence
by Randolph L. Lucente

The Recovery Philosophy and Direct Social Work Practice

Joseph Walsh

Virginia Commonwealth University

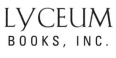

LYCEUM
BOOKS, INC.

Chicago, Illinois

© 2013 by Lyceum Books, Inc.

Published by

LYCEUM BOOKS, INC.
5758 S. Blackstone Ave.
Chicago, Illinois 60637
773+643-1903 fax
773+643-1902 phone
lyceum@lyceumbooks.com
www.lyceumbooks.com

Cover image © Cammeraydave | Dreamstime.com

6 5 4 3 2 1   13 14 15 16

ISBN 978-1-935871-23-1

Printed in the United States of America.

Library of Congress Cataloging-in-Publication Data

Walsh, Joseph (Joseph F.)
    The recovery philosophy and direct social work practice / Joseph Walsh.
        p. cm.
    ISBN 978-1-935871-23-1 (pbk. : alk. paper)
    1. Psychiatric social work. 2. Social work with people with mental disabilities.
3. Mentally ill—Services for. I. Title.
    HV689.W35   2013
    362.2′0425—dc23

                                                                    2012014684

To Kenny Weiss (1948–2012), my friend and mentor

Contents

Preface

The concept of recovery in mental health refers to an individual's personal journey toward wellness that involves developing, among other things, hope, secure material supports, a positive sense of self, supportive relationships, opportunities for social inclusion, and a sense of life purpose (Stotland, Mattson, & Bergeson, 2008). These goals have always been considered appropriate for persons who utilize mental health services, but recovery as a social development emphasizes as never before the person's self-determination and reliance on extraprofessional supports in achieving wellness. The recovery movement represents a major shift from a focus on symptom suppression to global health and development.

The profession of social work is uniquely situated to join with persons who experience mental illness in mutually developing strategies for their holistic recovery. Social workers have always understood that the quality of a person's functioning is dependent on the resources and supports available in the external environment. *The Recovery Philosophy and Direct Social Work Practice* explores the potential of the social work profession to operationalize its value base in helping persons with mental illnesses work toward recovery. The book addresses the ways that social workers can implement and support recovery activities through the following topics:

- The philosophy of recovery, with examples of its models
- A social work perspective on recovery and one specific model for professional practice
- The social worker–consumer relationship as the basis for recovery intervention
- Spiritual or existential issues in recovery
- Recovery practice with consumers who experience schizophrenia, depression, bipolar disorder, and autism spectrum disorders
- Endings in recovery practice
- The future of the recovery movement

Each of the four intervention chapters in Part 2 of the book includes consumer perspectives on the featured mental illness and extended examples of social workers and clients collaborating on recovery goals. Part 2 concludes with a chapter on ending interventions with recovering consumers, and a short final chapter considers the future of the recovery movement.

This book is targeted to social workers who provide individual, group, and family services to consumers in mental health and other social service agencies. It is not a program and policy book, but rather a practical guide for direct practitioners. Social workers who read this book will hopefully be better positioned to offer recovery-oriented services to persons with a variety of mental disorders in ways that are collaborative and that reflect a social, rather than medical, perspective on mental illness.

The Book's Organization

The Recovery Philosophy and Direct Social Work Practice is intended for use in both undergraduate- and graduate-level social work programs. It is suitable for the following types of courses:

- Clinical (or direct, or micro) social work practice.
- Clinical human behavior in the social environment, sometimes offered as a diagnostic or assessment course, often with a focus on the *Diagnostic and Statistical Manual of Mental Disorders* (American Psychiatric Association [APA], 2000).
- A variety of curriculum electives, such as, in the author's own school, social work practice in community mental health or social work practice in health care.

The book might also be of interest to practicing professionals who are eager to learn more about the recovery philosophy, a topic that may not have been covered when they were in school, and how they might incorporate it into their work.

The book is organized to build upon the social work profession's current knowledge and value base as a means of demonstrating how existing interventions can be expanded and adapted to more collaboratively work with consumers toward furthering their goals of holistic recovery from mental illness. The first three chapters of Part 1 set the stage for the profession's participation with recovering consumers by discussing definitions and several models of recovery. The next three chapters articulate the components of a specific social work model for recovery intervention. Part 2 of the book investigates how the intervention material already covered can be applied to work with consumers who face four major types of mental illness. The topic of autism spectrum disorders is included as an example of mental illness recovery that incorporates extensive social advocacy initiatives. It will be shown how the particular challenges persons with these types of mental illness face can be addressed with different sets of collaborative interventions. Each chapter will conclude with a summary of major chapter learning points and several questions for reflection or discussion.

It is my hope that readers of this book will become energized advocates for their clients with mental illnesses, and that this book provides them with new strategies for helping clients that will add to their own sense of professional mission.

A Note on Terminology

Throughout my practice career, persons with mental illnesses who receive professional services have been called "patients," "clients," and "consumers." For purposes of consistency, and recognizing that not all readers will agree with my choice of terms, I will refer to persons with mental illness as "persons" or "individuals" in a general context, and I will refer to them as "consumers" in the context of their receiving formal services.

Acknowledgments

I would like to recognize the following persons for their substantial assistance throughout my writing of this book: Carla Beck, Jacqueline Corcoran, Heather Dail, Ellen Hart, Brittany Leggett, Bonnie Neighbor, Shannon McNett, Renae Sands, Margaret Walsh, and Amy Wagner. I also want to thank the following reviewers of the first draft of the manuscript:

- Thomas Meenaghan, *New York University*
- Henry Kronner, *Aurora University*
- Patrick Konkin, *Vancouver Island University*
- Tuula Heinonen, *University of Manitoba*
- Daniel Salhani, *University of British Columbia*
- Lin Fang, *University of Toronto*
- Ronald John San Nicolas, *University of Washington, Tacoma*

Part 1

Social Work and the Recovery Philosophy

Chapter 1

Introduction: A Social Worker's Journey toward the Recovery Philosophy

As part of this introduction, I want to describe my own professional journey to recovery. Since I've been a practicing social worker for many years, it is fair to assume that I have not always been a proponent of this philosophy.

I've been a full- or part-time mental health professional for thirty-eight years, and a practicing social worker for thirty-three years. Throughout my career, I have primarily worked with persons who have chronic mental illnesses. My perspectives on working with these persons have evolved over the years. Of course, times are always changing with regard to social and professional perspectives on mental health and mental illness. Diagnostic categories, the various professions' attitudes about diagnosis, and wisdom about preferred interventions all change over time, although it may be wrong to assume that change always represents an advance. For example, although consumer rights with regard to involuntary hospitalization expanded during the 1970s, 1980s, and 1990s, some states have implemented new restrictions on those rights in the past ten years due to such events as the 2006 Virginia Tech shootings.

It is not my intention here to evaluate the quality of the developments in human services practice; rather, it is only my intention to emphasize that changes in service delivery are continuous. Because I am aware of those constant changes, I was offended fifteen years ago during a conversation I had with a doctoral student at my university. She was researching the benefits of clubhouse programs. The basic value of the clubhouse model is that all consumers, regardless of their level of disability, can contribute meaningfully to a shared community (Jackson, 2001). Clubhouses offer supportive relationships and opportunities, and include members in all aspects of group life in the promotion of work, education, and social relationships. During our conversation, the student stated her belief that these centers had only become widespread in the 1990s because, prior to that time, social workers and other professionals had been, in her words, "paternalistic," "opposed to client empowerment," and "operating from a distorted sense of values." I took issue with her comments, not least because I had been a social worker during those earlier decades and had always tried to provide quality care for my clients (the term "consumer" did not come into wide usage until the 1990s). When I suggested my perspective to the student, she replied, "Well, yes, you did try—you just didn't know any better at the time."

The student's comments implied that today we know how best to help persons with mental illnesses, but in previous decades we did not. Her perspective represented to me a false evolutionary perspective that sees the current situation as the most valid. I felt that her criticism was a disservice to the thousands of social workers over the years who have devoted their careers to doing the best work possible with their clients. Twenty years from now, it is likely that social workers will look back on today's practitioners with the same criticisms. In my opinion, it is not fair to judge practitioners retrospectively in this way, which brings me to the issue of the recovery philosophy of mental illness. How is it different from philosophies of mental health and mental illness that have gone before? I use my own story to describe what I see as the current context of the recovery movement.

I started out as a psychiatric technician, working the afternoon shift (2:30–11:00) at an esteemed private psychiatric hospital in the Midwest. Fresh out of college with a sociology degree, it was an inspiring, life-changing experience. I was considered to be a very good but low-ranking nursing staff member at the hospital. I worked on a unit of nineteen patients, as they were then called, facilitating informal social activities after they had completed their structured activities for the day. Mine was the long-term unit, where patients stayed for up to several years. Most of the patients had diagnoses of major mental illness. The unit staff included three psychiatrists: one was an analyst, another was a cognitive-behaviorist focused on helping patients emancipate, and a third was more focused on medication intervention. The unit also had a single social worker for family work, and a representative of the adjunctive therapy department who designed each patient's schedule of rehabilitation activities. A psychologist was available to perform psychological testing. Two nurses and two psychiatric technicians staffed each eight-hour shift on the unit. The prevailing wisdom of the time was that the major mental illnesses should be treated primarily with psychotherapy.

The famous social worker Herbert Strean (2002) once wrote that, in his opinion, the best therapists for persons with schizophrenia are first-year graduate students, because they don't know what schizophrenia is and treat these persons as people. This perspective pretty much characterized the work of the psychiatric technicians on my unit. Our job was to be present to manage behavior and engage the patients in constructive recreational activities. We spent much of our time during my evening shift organizing outdoor sports, and card and board games. The staff and the patients enjoyed each other's company. I remember being initially surprised that many patients who had schizophrenia seemed normal in so many ways. In fact, I mistook one such patient for a staff member during my orientation week. I was also struck by the fact that people with psychotic disorders could have such good senses of humor. I had thought that psychosis would jumble a person's thoughts so much that he or she wouldn't be able to understand humor.

It seemed to us (the psychiatric technicians) that patient life on the unit was as therapeutic as anything the doctors or activity therapists were doing—although no doubt the members of those other professions would disagree. We were told that the patients' therapy (thirty minutes, three times per week), activities (four per day, ninety minutes each), and family therapy sessions (every two weeks), along with the medications, were the keys to their recovery. The professional staff all agreed that success was to be measured by symptom amelioration and the patient's establishment of a conventional way of life, with or without other caregivers. Assuming that the other professionals knew best, we went about our business of developing positive, informal relationships with the patients. It appears in hindsight that the work we did was a kind of rough approximation of recovery practice.

Despite our companionable attitudes toward the patients, we believed in and supported some policies that would now be considered unethical. As examples, patients had no choices about the interventions they received. Voluntary patients could be held for ten days after their requests for discharge, giving staff time to consider pursuing their involuntary commitment. Patients were restricted from receiving or making phone calls and from routinely having visitors. They had to earn privileges to leave the unit without staff accompaniment. They could be forcibly escorted to a locked security room for unspecified periods if they engaged in dangerous acting-out behaviors. Patients had no access to their own records. Even the psychiatric technicians accepted that in most cases the staff always knew best, and that the patients' judgment was not as good as ours with regard to making many decisions for themselves.

These definitely were not the days of the recovery movement. Many staff had paternalistic attitudes toward the patients, who were presumed to have disorders that required intervention from experts. Still, I learned more than anything else that psychiatric patients were pretty much regular people with unique personalities and potentials. The work was interesting, fun, and rewarding, and I soon decided to develop a career in the human services. I decided on social work so that I could be a primary practitioner with the kinds of clients I had come to love, and I earned a master of social work (MSW) degree.

For the next fourteen years I was a clinical social worker and case manager at two community mental health centers in central Ohio. At the first agency, I was a member of the three-person geriatric evaluation team (services to older adults) for eighteen months, and was then transferred to the aftercare department (services to persons with serious mental illness) for the same duration. In both positions, I provided interventions including assessment, planning, counseling, crisis intervention, resource development, and linkage activities to housing, vocational rehabilitation, education, and day treatment centers for caseloads averaging thirty clients (as they were then called) in the first position and seventy-five clients in the second. Because most of the clients came to our offices for scheduled counseling sessions, our relationships tended to be more formal than in the hospital. I worked in both programs as part of an interdisciplinary team that included psychiatrists, nurses, and social workers. In the community I interacted with staff from psychiatric hospitals, nursing homes, and other human services agencies.

By the 1980s, psychiatric hospitals were considered to be overly restrictive and anachronistic from both human rights and therapeutic points of view. It was believed that most persons with serious mental illness could live successfully in the community if they had adequate personal and professional supports. State and federal policies were enacted to support this emphasis on community-based care. Although this principle of the least restrictive environment represented an advance from hospital care, social and professional attitudes about clients had not changed significantly. People with mental illnesses were still considered to be emotionally fragile, and not always aware of their own best interests. Social workers were inclined to assert a fair amount of control over their clients' lives. The administrators in my program reminded us that it was our responsibility to keep the clients safe, and that we needed to be careful not to have expectations that were "too high," because these might set clients up for failure.

With our degree of oversight in making linkages to other service agencies, clients remained quite dependent on us. Our supervisors promoted a principle of aggressive case management, and social workers were evaluated in large part on their abilities to keep clients out of psychiatric hospitals. We were discouraged from providing psychotherapy, since this had been "proven" not useful for clients with long-term psychotic disorders. Our time was to be spent securing safe living environments for clients above all else (and to make sure they took their medication).

I generally accepted these premises as valid, but also began reacting against what I saw as the controlling nature of case management. During my annual evaluations, I was credited with having good therapeutic skills, but I was encouraged to work with my clients more aggressively so that they would accept more of the formal community supports being made available to them, even though these were known to be of varying quality. I became frustrated with what I believed was a one-dimensional approach to working with clients: I thought there was a place for reflective and cognitive-behavioral therapies (CBTs) in working with them. Eventually I found a social work position at another agency that allowed me to develop my practice skills more broadly.

At the second community mental health agency (MHA), where I worked from the mid-1980s to the mid-1990s, I was given responsibility for coordinating the aftercare program, which is now known as the case management program. I provided direct services to a caseload of thirty clients and was responsible for community resource development, staff supervision, and staff development regarding interventions for clients with mental illnesses.

Most significant to my professional development, I learned how to be a therapist. The agency was well known at that time as being one of few in the county that focused on psychotherapy for all clients (now known as consumers), although to be fair the staff did not have much experience with persons who had psychotic disorders. I was surrounded by skilled practitioners and learned how to provide ego, object relations, and family systems approaches, among others, to clients. I had never been encouraged to be a therapist before and enjoyed developing those skills. I became more convinced than ever that psychotherapy could be effectively combined with traditional case management (and medication) activities when working with consumers who had mental illnesses. With this dual focus, I was able to know my clients intimately and help them work toward their personal goals while also helping them secure basic community living needs. Still, the agency was looked at with some suspicion by the county mental health planning board, because they considered us to be too traditional in how we worked with consumers. We expected consumers to come to the agency for services, much like private practice agencies, and we spent too little time being case managers.

During my ten years at the agency I developed two intervention groups: the Family Education and Support Group was the first program of its type in the region for families of those with a mental illness, and I was a founding member of the state's first Schizophrenics Anonymous self-help group. All of these activities reflected my love for persons with mental illness, and my focus expanded to include their families. If my work was paternalistic at times (mostly, in my view, by being overly cautious in keeping my consumers in a limited range of so-called safe environments), it also featured a collaborative, holistic focus that was moving me toward a recovery philosophy.

The mid-1980s represented the beginning of the social work profession's active strengths approach to working with consumers, but I still viewed them as being fragile, although less so than I had previously thought, and continued at times to facilitate involuntary hospitalizations and to make court appearances questioning the capacities of some consumers to care for their children. I also enjoyed acting as an expert in matters of treating mental illness. The agency psychiatrists encouraged medication use without much mutual consumer negotiation. Consumers had limited access to their records and could be refused all agency services if they refused any one of them.

My conversion to what later became known as a recovery philosophy was furthered in the late 1980s when the county funding body received a major foundation grant and announced that all agencies would be required to implement PACT (Program for Assertive Community Treatment) interventions. Persons with mental illness would be served by teams of five case managers providing around-the-clock availability. Psychotherapy, conceptualized as office-centered verbal treatment focused on the client's internal life, was not to be part of the intervention, however. It was believed that social workers were spending too much time in their offices providing unproductive therapy rather than being out in the community helping consumers meet their basic needs.

In response to this antitherapy mandate, I wrote a letter to the funding board, arguing for a clinical case management model of intervention whereby a single social worker would be responsible for consumer care in a holistic manner, including verbal therapies and case management. My proposal was rejected, however, and subsequently the employment credentials for agency case managers for PACT were lowered to require only a bachelor's degree in a helping profession. I believed this move was dehumanizing for consumers in its assumption that persons with mental illness did not merit highly trained social workers but my point of view was not endorsed by community mental health administrators.

While my agency was reorganizing its services to incorporate PACT, I began my doctoral studies in social work, keeping direct practice issues with persons who have mental illness at the forefront of my academic work. My doctoral dissertation supported the effectiveness of many elements of the PACT model, but also described its limitations in denying the potentially therapeutic elements of worker or consumer relationships.

I left full-time direct practice in 1993 after completing my Ph.D. and accepting a faculty position at my current university. I continued to provide direct services, however, on a part-time basis at various public agencies in the Richmond community. I volunteered at a variety of agencies serving persons with mental illness, leading support groups, and working with individual clients and their families. This is where my transformation to recovery-oriented practice reached its current position. For the first time in my career, I was a volunteer service provider, and as such was freed of many of the constraints that add pressure to the work of full-time social workers. I had a relatively small caseload and modest paperwork responsibilities, and as a licensed practitioner with many years of experience I was permitted much leeway in how I worked with consumers. Just as significantly, I had full access to the professional literature about the potential of a recovery perspective on mental illness.

In some ways, my work has come full circle, back to my days as a psychiatric technician, when I enjoyed interacting with consumers informally, having time to get to know them as well-rounded human beings with various aspirations. I've been reminded during this process that an employing organization's policies and procedures have great impact on the degree to which recovery principles can be incorporated into a social worker's interventions; fortunately, many mental health organizations are evolving in ways that are conducive to this practice. I don't believe I am by nature any better or worse as a social worker than I have ever been, or any less committed to the welfare of my consumers. Now, as always, I work with the best information I have at hand to be a resource for my consumers.

Chapter 2

The Recovery Philosophy of Mental Illness

> I see my life as a healing process, not as a mental illness. There are still days when I feel hopeless, depressed, and apathetic. I have not eliminated the chemistry of my humanity. The gamut of emotions is a human experience. I do not think of myself as someone with an illness, but I must address the imbalance. I maintain my self-care, psychiatry, exercise, proper nutrition, and connectedness with others. (Virginia Organization of Consumers Advocating Leadership [VOCAL], 2009, p. 129)

Recovery in mental health refers to a consumer's journey toward wellness and emphasizes his or her primary role and responsibility in achieving wellness. The recovery movement became prominent in the 1990s and represents a major transformative shift from a focus on symptom suppression to one of holistic health for persons with mental illness (White, Boyle, & Loveland, 2005). The purpose of this chapter is to consider definitions of recovery as a philosophy, or basic set of values and beliefs, for living. An awareness of these definitions will help orient social workers to their various possible roles in the consumer-driven process. Some specific models of recovery will be described in chapter 4.

Many people with serious mental illness identify themselves as normal people with certain disabilities or challenges. This stands in contrast to the prevailing focus of intervention in the Western world during the past half-century that has featured the eradication of symptoms and illness as the primary goal of the helping professions. That is, people with long-term disorders need not delay resuming a full life while waiting for their symptoms or illness to disappear, or to be "cured." The person can function well in spite of, or along with, his or her symptoms. Professional strategies to promote recovery can focus simultaneously on the individual and on his or her environment.

Inherent in recovery philosophy is the idea that mental illness, however it is described and defined, does not take over the entirety of a person, but exerts varying degrees of impact on specific domains of functioning. Mental illness leaves many domains of functioning intact, so consumers retain areas of health and competence alongside their problem areas. The person is always there and should be accorded all of his or her human rights and responsibilities. This is not to say that consumers always are allowed to choose their interventions, or that professionals do not sometimes decide what is best for them. The recovery philosophy does, however, value a consumer's right to self-determination as it extends into how he or she interacts with professionals. We will address inevitable controversies regarding self-determination throughout the book.

The current definition of mental disorder utilized by the American Psychiatric Association (2000, p. x) is a "significant behavioral or psychological syndrome or pattern that occurs in an individual and that is associated with present distress (e.g., a painful symptom) or disability (i.e., impairment in one or more important areas of functioning) or with significantly increased risk of suffering death, pain, disability, or an important loss of freedom." The syndrome or pattern "must not be an expectable and culturally sanctioned response to a particular event." Whatever its cause, "it must currently be considered a manifestation of behavioral, psychological, or biological dysfunction in the individual." Thus, mental illness resides within the person.

The above definition summarizes the APA's medical model of working with persons who have mental, emotional, and behavioral problems. The model, while useful in many ways, and representing a strongly institutionalized system of care, uses many criteria and definitions that are inconsistent with a recovery philosophy, and therefore is said by many critics to not promote a culture in which people with such problems can recover: "What a society labels to be 'mental illness' may be no more than a judgment, from a particular time and perspective, tinged with the preconceptions, needs, and fears of the culture doing the judging" (VOCAL, 2009, p. 11).

Definitions of Recovery

Recovery is a concept that has been defined in many ways during its relatively short life. There is a general philosophy of recovery as well as specific models of recovery. These models are guiding strategies for consumers to follow in their recovery processes, or for policy makers to follow in supporting recovery-oriented services. Not all these models are consistent with one another.

Part of the confusion over the meaning of the term "recovery" is that it can be understood as an outcome or a process. One dictionary defines recovery as "a return to an original state; a gradual healing (through rest) after sickness or injury, or the act of regaining or saving something lost (or in danger of becoming lost)" (Oxford Online Dictionary, 2012). This definition emphasizes a person's return to a previous level of health. The person has had an illness, but eventually overcomes it to return to "normal," as with a bodily infection. Another dictionary defines recovery as "the act, process, or an instance of recovering; the process of combating a disorder (as alcoholism) or a real or perceived problem" (Merriam-Webster's Online Dictionary, 2010). This definition implies that one's recovery is not necessarily a return to an original state; instead, recovery represents all efforts to deal with a condition as effectively as possible. The person may not return to what might be called normal, or to the pre-illness state, but he or she can make adjustments that facilitate optimal functioning in the presence of the illness. It is the latter definition that captures the spirit of recovery in mental health, except that the recovery philosophy recognizes that some consumers may transcend their pre-illness state in some ways.

With this distinction of two types of recovery, we can now consider several definitions of recovery in mental illness, the first few of which are offered by mental health professionals. According to the *Social Workers' Desk Reference*, recovery is "a process of developing individual potential and realizing life goals while surmounting the trauma and difficulties presented by behavioral, emotional, or physical challenges. For persons with a serious mental disorder, recovery involves a process of personal transformation in which the disorder becomes less central in a person's life as he or she achieves outcomes that increasingly bring personal meaning and life satisfaction" (Roberts, 2009, p. 1203).

The Center for Psychiatric Rehabilitation, which has been instrumental in promoting the recovery movement, defines the term as "a deeply personal, unique process of changing one's attitudes, values, feelings, goals, skills, and roles. It is a way of living a satisfying, hopeful, and contributing life even with limitations caused by the illness. Recovery involves the development of new meaning and purpose in one's life as one grows beyond the catastrophic effects of mental illness" (Anthony, 1993, p. 11).

Larry Davidson, one of the foremost human service professionals writing on the topic, defines mental health recovery as "the person's assumption of increasing control over his or her psychiatric condition while claiming responsibility for his or her own life. Recovery remains possible even though a person's condition may not change; it involves some component of acceptance of illness" (Davidson, O'Connell, Tondora, Lawless, & Evans, 2005, p. 485).

Some state departments of mental health have adopted the recovery philosophy as a guiding policy framework. As one example, the Ohio Department of Mental Health (ODMH) (2011) defines recovery as "a personal process that involves overcoming the negative impact of a psychiatric disability despite its continued presence. In a recovery-oriented system, mental health consumers rebuild meaningful lives while receiving services that enable them to recover and decrease their dependence on the system." It strives to "provide education and technical support for recovery programs and/or activities that reach beyond the critical issues of assuring personal safety and managing symptoms and focus on the rebuilding of full, productive lives despite a mental disorder."

The Substance Abuse and Mental Health Services Administration (SAMHSA) of the federal government convened a National Consensus Conference on Mental Health Recovery and Mental Health Systems Transformation in 2003 that included both professionals and consumers, among other participants. Participants developed the following consensus statement on recovery: "Mental health recovery is a journey of healing and transformation enabling a person with a mental health problem to live a meaningful life in a community of his or her choice while striving to achieve his or her full potential" (SAMHSA, 2006).

At its core, recovery can be understood less as a specific model for living, and more as a philosophy or attitude, one that encourages consumers to acquire or regain personal power and a valued place in their communities, often, but not always, with the assistance of mental health professionals. Recovery is commonly addressed in the context of a social disability paradigm rather than a medical one. Within this paradigm, recovery refers to a person's right and ability to have a safe, dignified, and meaningful life in the community of his or her choice, despite continuing disability resulting from the illness (Beecher, 2009; Reindal, 2008).

The recovery philosophy can be addressed at three transformational levels (Bonnie Neighbor, Advocacy Coordinator, VOCAL, personal communication, May 2011). At the systems level, state and federal policy makers may enact mandates for programs that incorporate a recovery perspective. At the community level, consumers and professionals may institute programs and develop resources to create supports that are not available in the formal service system. At the personal level, consumers assume greater power to direct their own lives (and interventions); at the spiritual level, they work to make sense of their conditions in ways that go beyond what is emphasized in the medical model.

There tend to be differences in how recovery is conceptualized among professionals and consumers (Davidson, Harding, & Spaniol, 2006). These differences derive from the vantage point of those persons or groups offering the definition. For example, some consumers might even argue against the existence of mental illness, or propose a very different conceptualization from that of professionals. Somewhat paradoxically, the recovery movement has been consumer generated, but is currently embraced by many human services professionals, who inevitably bring some limits to its implementation.

Professional (or clinical) approaches tend to focus on observable improvements in consumer symptoms and social functioning, and on the role of professional intervention. Consumer (sometimes called rehabilitation) models tend to emphasize peer support, empowerment, and the primacy of personal experience. There is a stronger focus on life meaning within the context of a supposedly enduring disability. Furthermore, many recovering consumers do not accept the legitimacy of psychiatric diagnostic labels, which many believe to be dehumanizing and reductionistic.

The Loner

Anita Flores was a twenty-five-year-old single Latina woman living with her younger sister in a condominium owned by their father. Anita had experienced schizophrenia for the past six years and appeared in the eyes of her social worker to be barely functional. She had no contact with anyone in her large city of residence other than her sister, father, and social worker (whom she visited reluctantly). Anita liked to take walks, but appeared to be lost in her thoughts and rarely spoke. She rarely bathed or showered, and ate only intermittently. Anita had been involuntarily hospitalized several times by her father, and only agreed to see the social worker at his urging.

Anita was assigned to work with a skilled agency practitioner who managed to develop enough of a relationship with her that they could have brief conversations. But Anita was clear that she did not have a mental disorder. "There is nothing wrong with me mentally," she stated. "I have problems like everyone, but only about planning my day so I can get my walk in. Don't start talking to me about mental illness or drugs or I won't come back." Anita had dropped out of treatment several times before for that very reason, so the social worker respected her wish. During their meetings, he always spoke to her about managing the various challenges of her modest lifestyle. Interestingly, she eventually agreed to take medications so that she might feel less tense.

Recovery, then, involves consumers accepting and owning their disabilities, however they understand them; developing their own goals; and making their own decisions about the types of formal and informal services they wish to receive. They often prefer to view health-care professionals as partners rather than authorities in assessment, goal setting, and choosing intervention modalities. With their lives focused on recovery, people with mental illnesses do not perceive themselves to be so much clients of human service professionals as they are persons with certain limiting characteristics who can lead productive and gratifying lives with a partial reliance on professionals. Perhaps most important, recovery is not just about finding a new way of surviving in the external world, but also about finding a new way of understanding one's internal world (Deegan, 1996).

Because mental health service consumers have been at the forefront of the recovery movement, it is especially worth hearing what they say about the concept. All but one of the following quotes was selected from consumers featured in the book *Firewalkers* (VOCAL, 2009).

Western medicine sees mental health symptoms as a problem to be stamped out, and doesn't see the holistic picture: there is something off balance that needs to be gently righted, not medicated out of existence. If you think of one piece of a person as having to be medicated out of existence, you may be blunting them of their other gifts. (VOCAL, 2009, p. 11)

I don't think much of the world appreciates the intensity of the internal struggle associated with mental illness—the way it can destroy relationships, vocational success, hopes, dreams. Being able to come through this with a realization that life isn't over, that there are still things worth living and fighting for, requires incredible resilience. It's a resilience that you wouldn't know you had unless you found that you could indeed make it through the fire. (VOCAL, 2009, p. 66)

I changed my relationship with mental health providers. I began to look at people who were providing treatment for me as co-partners instead of people trying to tell me what to do. I took their advice into consideration and then made my own choice about what's best for me. I began to direct my own treatment. (VOCAL, 2009, p. 151)

Hope of knowing that everything that is, that I go through, would not continue the rest of my life, that there would be an end of it; and just knowing that I knew that, I could keep going. (Davidson, Borg, Marin, Topor, Mezzina, & Sells, 2005, p. 184)

The Fundamental Values of Recovery

While there are many definitions of recovery, several of which are presented above, the process always incorporates certain fundamental values. The following consensus values have been articulated by SAMHSA (2006). Clearly there are conflicts at times in how social workers operationalize these values, and these points of disagreement will be addressed throughout this book.

- Hope is the catalyst of the recovery process. Recovery provides the essential message of a better future, that consumers can overcome the obstacles confronting them as they pursue psychological growth. As already noted, research has shown that many more consumers with mental illness can achieve their recovery goals, or even exceed them, than was assumed for many years. A consumer's sense of hope is best when internalized, but peers, families, friends, and providers can foster its development and help to maintain it.
- Self-direction. Consumers can lead, control, exercise choice over, and determine their own path of recovery by optimizing their autonomy, independence, and control of material and emotional

resources. When working with professionals, consumers should participate in making decisions about services they will utilize. It is the self, not the service professional, who is the agent of recovery.

- Individualized action. There are multiple pathways to recovery based on each consumer's unique strengths, needs, preferences, experiences, and cultural background. Consumers should not assume that any particular practices (including evidence-based practices, which will be discussed later) are necessary for their recovery.

- Empowerment. Consumers should retain the authority to choose from a range of recovery options and participate in all decisions, professional and otherwise, that will affect their lives. Through empowerment, consumers gain control of their destinies and can influence the institutions that affect their lives. Empowerment models of recovery emphasize that disabling conditions are not necessarily permanent, and that other consumers who have recovered can be role models by sharing their experiences, both their successes and their failures. There are limits to social workers' abilities to facilitate consumer empowerment, as evidenced in the following example.

A Bad Temper

Keith was a physically imposing twenty-five-year-old man with severe recurrent depressive episodes and low self-esteem. He had long ago learned to use his size and angry outbursts as a means of intimidating others, acting out his feelings of inferiority, and getting his way. One day, Keith walked into the agency without an appointment and demanded to see his social worker. When the receptionist said this would not be possible because his social worker was busy with another client, Keith exploded at her in full view of others in the waiting room, screaming profanities and making physical threats against her. The terrified receptionist ran from the room, and Keith's social worker, hearing the commotion, came out of his office to confront the client. A shouting match ensued, after which the social worker ordered Keith out of the agency. He finally complied, but was banned from the agency property as a result of the incident. The social worker only agreed to meet with Keith in public places afterwards, and he rarely agreed to accompany the client on community outings.

- Holism. Recovery encompasses a consumer's entire life, including the mind, body, spirit, and community. It attends to such areas as housing, employment, education, mental health, other health-care services, spirituality, creativity, social networks, community participation, and family supports.
- Nonlinearity. Recovery is not a step-by-step growth process: it can include setbacks. Recovery begins with one's awareness that positive change in life is possible, along with the knowledge that life is an uncertain journey. Furthermore, recovery can continue even if symptoms recur because recovery changes the frequency, duration, and experience of symptoms.
- Strengths basis. Recovery focuses on valuing and building on one's capacities, resiliencies, talents, coping abilities, and inherent worth. It focuses on wellness, not illness. Consumers can leave their old, limiting roles behind and engage in new life roles that do not necessarily involve adherence to the expectations of others, including those of professional helpers.
- Peer support. Recovery requires other people who believe in and stand by the person in recovery. Mutual support, including the sharing of experiential knowledge and skills with other consumers, is essential to one's recovery. The stories of other consumers are as valuable as professional intervention. Consumers can provide each other with a sense of belonging and support, and a range of valued roles.
- Respect. Recovery involves overcoming the effects of being identified as a psychiatric patient. That is, the consumer needs to transcend the social stigma attached to mental illness, a stigma that at times may be perpetuated by professionals. Community acceptance, which includes protecting consumers' rights and eliminating discrimination, is critical to the recovery process. Self-acceptance and a belief in one's self are vital. It is important to state that it is not just possible for recovering consumers to make a contribution to their communities: they already do so, as human beings. Peer support can be an essential source of respect, including the activities of advocacy groups.

- Responsibility. Consumers have personal responsibility for their self-care and recovery journeys. They make choices for themselves that involve risks, some that will be productive and others that may lead to setbacks. Consumers, like anyone else, have the right to fail as well as to succeed in their efforts.

Several additional principles of recovery have been emphasized from the perspective of professionals involved in psychiatric rehabilitation services, including (Onken, Craig, Ridgway, Ralph, & Cook, 2007):

- Recovery can occur without professional intervention, although many consumers accept such assistance.
- There is no necessary correlation between one's recovery potential and mental health history.
- Recovery from the consequences of a psychiatric condition, including stigma, is often more difficult than recovery from its symptoms.
- Significant recovery does not mean the person was never psychiatrically disabled.

A third set of recovery principles is offered by White and colleagues (2005) and is excerpted here (to avoid repetition with the above material):

- Treatment and recovery are not the same. Treatment refers to the ways professionals intervene to stabilize or alter the course of an illness, whereas recovery refers to the personal experiences of individuals as they move out of illness and into lives of greater health and wholeness.
- Recovery exists on a continuum of improved health and functioning. The mental health professions have long affirmed the concept of partial recovery, but consumers tend to reject the implicit limitations in this perspective and to consider holistic recovery as an ongoing process with no predictable end point.
- Recovery occurs at a different pace along the dimensions of physical, intellectual, emotional, relational, and personal functioning. Symptom recovery is not a singular, catch-all concept: consumers may experience growth in certain aspects of their lives, which in turn may promote growth in others. For example, improvements in cognitive functioning may promote enhanced vocational func-

tioning, while mood stabilization may enhance interpersonal functioning.

- Language is important to personal recovery. The use of certain types of language when referring to a consumer's status can have demoralizing effects on a recovering consumer and retard the process, while more positive language can facilitate hope and a constructive orientation to change. The ability of consumers to avoid internalizing terms that may be demeaning or limiting to them, and to select words that more accurately describe their experiences and aspirations, is critical. Examples of negative terms include illness, disability, disorder, deficit, remission, diagnosis, chemical imbalance, and symptoms. Examples of recovery-oriented terms include challenge, strengths, resilience, and goals.

A major theme in recovery is that consumers attend to the process quite differently. In an effort to get a sense of common recovery themes among consumers from several countries, a group of researchers conducted in-depth interviews with twelve consumers with long-term psychotic disorders from Italy, Norway, Sweden, and the United States (Davidson, Borg, et al., 2005). From their content analysis of responses, the researchers identified the following common themes:

- Consumers are determined to get better, establish a greater degree of self-control, and engage in an ongoing struggle to achieve a normal life.
- Consumers share a need for basic material resources and a sense of home, and they prioritize goals related to going out into the larger society and engaging in normal activities.
- Consumers struggle with issues related to the benefits and costs of medication, and the extent of their participation in mutual support and psychosocial interventions.
- Consumers strive to be accepted, as all people do, and to accept themselves as normal people who exist beyond their psychoses.
- Consumers routinely struggle with the effects of stigma and discrimination, having their rights respected, and returning to meaningful social roles through work and positive relationships outside the formal mental health system.

While recovery is very much with us, it has only been prominent for a decade or so. The question, "How did it emerge?" is answered next.

The Emergence of the Recovery Philosophy

This is a book about social work practice, so what follows is not intended to be an exhaustive review of social trends. Rather, it is a brief overview of how the consumer-driven recovery philosophy emerged in the United States and around the world.

Until recently, disability policy in the United States was based rather strictly on a medical model of care, which asserts that when people develop conditions that are abnormal or represent deviant physical processes they should receive the rehabilitative expertise of health-care professionals to return to normalcy, or as close to normalcy as possible (Beecher, 2009). "Patients" were not routinely encouraged to select from among the range of possible intervention options because professionals were considered to be the experts in those matters. As more people have become involved in advocacy efforts for persons with disabilities, however, a new social (recovery) model of disability has evolved, incorporating a central belief that the experiences of people with disabilities, rather than the preferences of those with professional expertise, should be a critical element in determining interventions as well as programs and policies (Reindal, 2008). This approach emphasizes self-advocacy and a belief that a society's resources and opportunities should be at times altered to better accommodate persons with disabilities, rather than trying to always fit people with disabilities into existing social structures. Among its implications, the social model of disability suggests that mental illness is not a disabling condition per se, but that the problem lies largely in how society treats people with mental illness.

How did this shift come about? Exhibit 2.1 includes a list of some major trends over the years in the United States that supported the emergence of the recovery philosophy (Dail, 2010). While in this book we generally only refer as far back as the 1950s, it is interesting to note that in the 1940s a group of discharged psychiatric patients in New York City formed an organization known as We Are Not Alone, with the goal of helping other patients transition from psychiatric hospitals to community life. Their efforts led to the development of Fountain House in 1948, a well-known psychosocial program located in that city that is a model for hundreds of other clubhouses that have come into being in the past thirty years. Among its principles are that members function as

---

Exhibit 2.1:   The Emergence of the Recovery Philosophy

History of self-help movements in the United States (such as
   Alcoholics Anonymous)

1940s
   • We Are Not Alone and Fountain House
1950s
   • Deinstitutionalization
1960s
   • The Community Mental Health Centers Act
   • Disability, gay, and civil rights
   • Women's liberation
1970s
   • The International Pilot Study of Schizophrenia
   • The psychiatric rehabilitation intervention outcome studies
   • Published personal stories of recovery
1980s
   • Increased numbers of peer-run services and clubhouses
   • Research that demonstrates effectiveness and efficacy of peer-
     run services
   • First statewide consumer conference (held in California)
1990s
   • Shared dissatisfaction with case management
   • Increased consumer leadership initiatives
   • Positions for consumers incorporated into conventional mental
     health services
2000s
   • The New Freedom Commission on Mental Health and the Fed-
     eral Action Agenda on Mental Health

---

equals with staff, are encouraged to pursue recovery in their own ways,
and are not there to receive formal mental health services.

For more than fifty years, the prevailing public policy in the United
States and Canada for the care of persons with serious mental illness has
been deinstitutionalization, with the goal of supporting consumers in
normal community settings as opposed to institutions (Mechanic,
2008). For the first forty of those fifty years, socially sanctioned responsibility for the care of those consumers rested with the mental health
professions (psychiatry, psychology, social work, nursing, and others),
most of which adhered to the medical model of intervention. It was

assumed that consumers experienced overwhelming social functioning deficits due to the severe nature of their disorders and thus required the assistance of expert professionals to make successful transitions to community living.

During the transition from hospital to community care in the 1970s, a new type of mental health practitioner, the case manager, emerged, represented by several of the helping professions, with social work prominent among them. Case managers focused their work in communities, where shelter, housing, and other basic consumer needs were met through existing but fragmented services such as the family, charities, Medicaid, Social Security, MHAs, and other public programs. Case managers made referrals and provided linkages to persons with mental illness in an effort to establish conventional lifestyles for them. Unfortunately, because of a lack of adequate support services many consumers experienced homelessness, poverty, unemployment, overmedication, and social discrimination, and they rotated in and out of residential facilities. Case managers did their best to provide quality care, but there was a shared dissatisfaction with the quality of life achieved by consumers in the formal service system, for the following reasons:

- Consumers were placed in living environments with insufficient social and psychological supports.
- There was an erroneous assumption that consumers would be accepted in their communities, and that stigma would eventually vanish.
- The focus on material supports produced a professional backlash against interventions (verbal therapies) that focused on the consumer's sense of self.

The major impetus for the recovery concept with regard to psychiatric disorders in the United States came from the consumer/survivor/ex-patient movement, a grassroots self-help and advocacy initiative that emerged during the 1980s (Davidson, Flanagan, Roe, & Styron, 2006). This movement was fueled by three factors. First was the published results of the International Pilot Study of Schizophrenia launched by the World Health Organization, the findings of which began to appear in the professional literature in the 1970s. These studies (summarized by Calabrese & Corrigan, 2005) demonstrated a broad heterogeneity in outcome for persons with serious mental illness. Indeed, partial to full recovery was observed in 25 to 65 percent of each sample, recovery being defined as "amelioration of symptoms and other deficits associated with the disorder to a sufficient degree that they no longer interfere with daily functioning, allowing the person to resume personal, social, and vocational activities within what is considered a normal range" (Calabrese & Corrigan, p. 73). There was also a growing professional literature in the 1980s, particularly in the psychiatric rehabilitation field, that provided positive evidence of intervention outcomes, again indicating that the course of the serious mental illnesses was more diverse than previously believed. Finally, as the consumer movement grew, there was a cumulative influence of published personal stories of recovery that added to these positive findings. In short, many people with serious mental illness recovered to a significant extent.

With this new understanding of the adaptive capacities of persons with mental illness, federal programs such as the National Institute of Mental Health's (NIMH) community support system policy in 1979 attempted to mobilize resources to better facilitate the movement of discharged consumers through their communities toward higher levels of independent living (Longhofer, Kubek, & Floersch, 2010). While constructive in many ways, this movement proved to be flawed because it continued to give priority to consumers receiving basic material needs rather than to their emotional well-being.

During the last two decades of the twentieth-century, policy makers and administrators sought to standardize case management practices to meet growing demands for provider accountability (Walsh, 2000). There continued to be an emphasis on basic needs and a shift away from psychological quality of life, however, because observable behavior was more easily measured than mental or emotional status. This ongoing focus on material resource development eventually presented service providers with a major problem: while the goal of case management was to promote independent living, few intervention models addressed aspects of the consumer's internal world that should be developed toward that end. Case managers, many of whom had modest professional credentials, lacked expertise in theories of human behavior and intervention that could account for variations in how consumers thought, acted, and felt. Case managers did not possess sufficient knowledge about how to stimulate and maintain consumer self-direction, responsibility, hope, and recovery. Furthermore, doing for rather than doing with had been a guiding principle of case management. The excesses of doing for negatively affected what would become a significant predictor of recovery: continuous and stable consumer relationships with both formal and informal caregivers.

Slowly, for the reasons described earlier, the recovery movement moved from the margins into the mainstream of self-help and professional intervention in the late 1990s. Its onset marked a significant conceptual shift toward the identification of client self-direction in all recovery processes. Recovery was adopted as the overarching aim of public mental health policy and practice in the 1999 "Report on Mental Health of the Surgeon General" (Davidson, O'Connell, et al., 2005). In the follow-up New Freedom Commission on Mental Health and the Federal Action Agenda on Mental Health, recovery was said to be the most important goal for the mental health service delivery system (U.S. Department of Health and Human Services Administration, Center for Mental Health Services, 2001).

President Bush's New Freedom Commission proposed transforming the mental health system in the United States by shifting the focus of care from traditional medical psychiatric treatment toward the concept of recovery, the impact of which was also felt in Canada. The New Freedom Commission advocated for the development of national and state initiatives to empower consumers and support recovery, with specific committees assigned to

- Launch nationwide pro-recovery, antistigma education campaigns;
- Develop and synthesize recovery policies;
- Train consumers in carrying out evaluations of mental health systems; and
- Further the development of peer-run services.

Currently, SAMHSA funds a limited number of state initiatives to help transform its systems toward a recovery focus, although it has directed all states to use their federal block grants for such transformative activities. Some states, including Ohio, Virginia, Wisconsin, and others, have redesigned their mental health systems to emphasize recovery values (Jacobson & Greenley, 2001). Similar initiatives are occurring in other countries, including Australia, Canada, England, and Israel (Ramon, Shera, Healy, Lachman, & Renouf, 2009). Each of these countries is emphasizing different aspects of recovery within its overall commitment to a recovery paradigm. Some put primary effort into making formal services more recovery oriented, some emphasize the development of supportive community resources and opportunities, and others fund consumer and peer alternatives.

Mental health service providers wishing to embrace a recovery perspective need to consider a number of challenging issues, such as these:

- What aspects of prevailing practice should be transformed?
- What alternative kinds of relationships with consumers should be established?
- How can recovery practitioners survive the inevitable disapproval from some professionals?
- How can consumers maintain ownership of recovery concepts while engaging in professional intervention and policy making?

A central component of the transformation process is the inclusion and partnership of people with serious mental illness in research, intervention, and policy enterprises. Within this context, mental health interventions are to be judged in terms of their efficacy in reducing the effects of mental illness as well as in promoting consumers' abilities to engage in the kinds of activities that appeal to them.

In summary, it is still a matter of debate whether the social model of disability policy best serves the needs of persons with mental illness (Reindal, 2008). Reliance on the medical model, for example, might lead to more resources being devoted to uncovering the causes of mental illness and its treatment. Perhaps the best development in social policy would be to promote both the medical and the social models of mental illness. Consumers would be able to select from a variety of interventions, and a combination of public and private resources would ensure access to those services. At the same time, society would begin to understand its need to embrace the perspectives and lifestyles of all individuals, including those with mental illness.

Controversial Issues in Recovery

Because recovery is a consumer-driven movement, and is sometimes at odds with prevailing practices, conflicts often emerge between recovery-minded consumers and professional treatment providers. These often center on boundary differences between consumer choice and professional treatment priorities in helping practices. The fields of psychiatry, psychology, and (yes) social work have traditionally controlled both the nature of and consumer access to certain interventions and support resources.

Concerns raised by many human services professionals about the recovery perspective are as follows (Davidson, O'Connell, Tondora, Styron, & Kangas, 2006):

- A focus on recovery may add to the burden of already stretched providers when it requires the addition of new resources.
- Recovery can happen only after, and as a result of, professional intervention.
- Much recovery-oriented professional care is neither reimbursable nor evidence based in nature.
- Recovery-oriented care devalues the role of professional intervention.
- Consumer choice increases providers' exposure to risk and liability.
- The recovery philosophy fails to recognize the difficulty of consumer empowerment, given the existing structure of social institutions.

Consumers' own concerns about the activities of mental health providers include the following:

- The language of consumerism may be used as a rhetorical device to reinforce the position of professionals.
- Professional power may be exercised by limiting the range of decisions that consumers make and by shaping roles to create the acceptance of expert authority.
- Support for consumerism may represent an off-loading of responsibility from the service provider to clients.
- The recovery philosophy might unfairly assume that all consumers can fully recover from mental illness, and thereby stigmatize those who do not.

A major issue in relationships between recovering consumers and helping professionals is, Who decides what is best for the consumer? Clearly, social workers are bound by their value systems to prevent their clients from engaging in behaviors that may be harmful to the self or others. The tensions that arise from this issue, and the socially sanctioned power differential between the two parties, will be acknowledged and addressed throughout this book.

One point of difference between many consumers and many providers is their attitudes toward evidence-based practice (EBP) interventions, a subject to which we now turn.

Evidence-Based Practice

It has become imperative in the past few decades for social workers to be able to demonstrate their practice effectiveness (Zlotnik, 2007). The profession's movement toward EBP is related to an increased need for accountability to consumers and third-party payers, and a desire to further the knowledge base of the profession. Put simply, the social worker is faced with answering the question, "What evidence do I have that a proposed intervention will be effective with my client?" Available practice guidelines are intended to provide social workers with organized knowledge in reaching relevant outcomes.

The systematic process of EBP emerged as a value in the medical fields during the 1990s, and involved professionals relying on research-based evidence to assess people for the presence of physical and mental disorders and determining how they might best respond to interventions (Sackett, Richardson, Rosenberg, & Haynes, 1997). This process of establishing generalizable research knowledge for treating persons with particular mental disorders required practitioners to formulate specific questions about intervention, locate relevant studies, and assess their credibility when deciding how to work with consumers. EBP meant that research studies justified a certain treatment approach for most or all consumers with a particular disorder. The following hierarchical model in EBP includes seven levels of knowledge, from most to least rigorous (Rosenthal, 2004):

1. Meta-analysis (a set of statistical methods for combining quantitative results from multiple studies to produce an overall summary of empirical knowledge on a given topic)
2. Systematic reviews (a comprehensive synthesis of the research that bears on a particular question, using organized and replicable procedures)
3. Well-designed individual experimental studies

4. Well-defined quasi-experimental studies
5. Well-designed nonexperimental studies
6. Series of case reports or expert committee reports with critical appraisal
7. Opinions of respected authorities based on clinical experiences

All human service professionals wish to engage in effective practice, but efforts to utilize EBP models are controversial among social workers and consumers for several reasons (Beutler & Baker, 1998; Chambless, 1998; Rosenthal, 2004). Most research methodologies have not yet been able to examine worker and consumer relationship factors in intervention, which are considered fundamental in many theories and among most consumers (Miller, Duncan, & Hubble, 2005). The personal characteristics of social workers are often overlooked, such as their relationship-development experience with various types of consumers and overall competence in carrying out particular interventions. Qualitative researchers—who focus on relatively few participants, but in greater depth—are also distrustful of efforts to generalize intervention outcomes because of the complexities inherent in every instance of clinical intervention (Davidson, 2003). Furthermore, reliance on intervention manuals, which are written directives used in many research studies, may limit the natural responsiveness of practitioners to unique aspects of clinical situations.

Perhaps most important, consumers do not agree that diagnostic categories are precise in capturing the essence of a consumer's life situation. Social workers must be cautious in assuming that any two consumers are alike, even if they share the same diagnostic label. Variables such as a person's social supports, socioeconomic status, distress level, motivation, intelligence, and other characteristics may be more important predictors of intervention response than a diagnosis. Some social workers thus believe that a reliance on EBP is reductionistic, simplifying the personality of the client, not accounting for differing skill levels of practitioners, and attempting to simplify the range of interventions that a practitioner actually provides (Miller et al., 2005).

The tensions between those who follow and are skeptical of the findings of EBP may represent a misunderstanding of the EBP concept, and in fact recovery and EBP orientations are not necessarily opposed to one another. While a strict adherence to empirically supported treatments does involve consulting lists of interventions rank-ordered by their research effectiveness, EBP is far more holistic in nature. In fact, Thyer and Pignotti (2011) argue that EBP requires a social worker's integration of best research evidence along with the social worker's clinical expertise and collaborative attention to the consumer's values. The term "best research evidence" refers to clinically relevant research, often from the basic sciences but especially from consumer-centered research. "Clinical expertise" refers to the social worker's reliance on his or her accumulated skills to assess each consumer's unique health state and the risks and benefits of potential interventions. "Consumer values" refers to the unique preferences and expectations that each consumer brings to the professional encounter. Regehr and Glancy (2010) add that the EBP process should include the social worker's attention to agency mandates and constraints, and the strengths and limitations of the broader resource environment. The EBP process does not represent the medical model because it does not suggest that human problems have a biological etiology, that problems are best addressed through biologically based interventions, or that medical professionals should be the primary providers of care. Furthermore, the systematic literature reviews used in EBP are not recommendations about what social workers should or should not do, but instead provide summaries of what the research has to say about an intervention.

Proponents of the recovery philosophy believe that professional intervention should always be tailored to the unique characteristics and goals of the consumer, and that such interventions cannot be generalized. Most consumers acknowledge that the perspectives of professionals and laypersons should be taken into account in developing research agendas so that unique issues of resources, service access, and consumer and organizational cultures are all considered.

Summary

The recovery movement represents a major shift in the treatment and rehabilitation of persons with mental illnesses, moving priority in decision making away from the professional provider and toward the consumer. While an overarching philosophy of recovery can be articulated, the ways in which that philosophy is operationalized among professionals and consumers in models of recovery are quite varied. Within the consumer-driven philosophy of recovery, the perceived roles of mental health professionals may be extensive or limited, or may change as the consumer moves along his or her recovery path. There is always the possibility of conflict between consumers and professionals in addressing recovery processes, which often reflects a difference between the two groups in perceived knowledge (including judgment), power, and expertise. In the next chapter, we will see that the values of the recovery philosophy have much in common with the values of the social work profession, and that practicing social workers have an opportunity to partner with consumers toward their goals of self-determination and satisfactory social functioning.

Major Chapter Learning Points

- Recovery represents the journey of a person with mental illness toward holistic (bio-psycho-social-spiritual) wellness, and emphasizes his or her primary role and responsibility in achieving wellness.
- The major impetus for the recovery movement in the United States has come from the consumer/survivor/ex-patient movement.
- Recovery philosophy can be addressed at three levels: the systems (state and federal policies), community (programs and resources), and personal (consumers assuming greater power to direct their own lives and to make sense of their conditions in ways that go beyond the medical model).
- Ten guiding values have been articulated to capture the essence of the recovery philosophy.
- Conflicts often emerge between recovery-minded consumers and professional treatment providers due to differing perspectives on consumer choices and professionals' priorities in helping practices.
- Although the growing allegiance to EBP among human service professionals seems dehumanizing to some consumers, it can be a collaborative process in developing individualized recovery plans.

Questions for Reflection or Discussion

1. Think about whether, in your own practice, interventions are focused on consumer recovery as a process or as an outcome. How would your work be organized differently if you worked from one perspective or the other?

2. To what extent do you believe that the fundamental values of recovery are realistic in today's social services environment? What are their limitations, if any?

3. Consider some possible issues that might arise in working with a client where you might feel compelled to overrule his or her goals or activities. How would you try to resolve any discrepancy?

4. How do you select interventions to use with persons who have mental illnesses? Do you consult the literature, rely on the expert opinions of others, or rely on your own experiential knowledge? If you rely on the judgment of peers or supervisors, on what do they base their own preferences?

Chapter 3

Social Work Practice and the Recovery Philosophy

People who gave me grace rather than judgment ultimately made the biggest difference in my life. (VOCAL, 2009, p. 63)

As described in the previous chapter, the recovery philosophy calls for a service environment in which consumers have primary or collaborative control over decisions about their own care. Helping consumers achieve their goals in this way is consistent with the values of the social work profession, which is committed to the empowerment and self-determination of all populations, particularly those who are traditionally disenfranchised. The purpose of this chapter is to describe how the social work profession is well situated to act in partnership with recovering consumers who have mental illnesses.

Most of the interventions used by direct social work practitioners are used as much by members of other helping professions. The manner in which these interventions are used may differ among professional groups, however, depending on the people served, the practice setting, and, most important, the value perspective of the profession. In fact, it is sometimes said that professions are distinguished more by their value bases than by any other defining characteristics (Dolgoff, Loewenberg, & Harrington, 2009).

It is important for social workers to consider how they can utilize the material presented in the upcoming chapters in ways that are true to their professional mission. In this chapter, we will review several defining characteristics of the social work profession and consider how consistent they are with the recovery philosophy of mental illness. We will consider the value base of social work practice, strengths-oriented social work practice, a risk and protective framework for social work practice, multiculturalism, consumer empowerment, and spirituality in recovery practice.

Defining Direct Social Work Practice

Direct, also called clinical, social work practice can be defined in a variety of ways. The definition presented here, developed by the author and other faculty at Virginia Commonwealth University's School of Social Work, represents an effort to capture the profession's broad scope:

> Direct social work practice is the application of social work theory and methods to the resolution and prevention of psychosocial problems experienced by individuals, families, and groups. These problems may include challenges, disabilities, or impairments, including mental, emotional, and behavioral disorders. Direct practice is grounded in the values of the social work profession and, as such, promotes social and economic justice by empowering consumers who experience oppression or vulnerability to problem situations. Direct practice is based on an application of human development theories within a psychosocial context, focused on issues of human diversity and multiculturalism. Social workers help consumers to enact psychological and interpersonal change, increase their access to social and economic resources, and maintain their achieved capacities and strengths. Assessment always incorporates the impact of social and political systems on consumer functioning. Interventions may include therapeutic, supportive, educational, and advocacy activities.

With this working definition in hand, we can now more fully consider the concepts of values, strengths, risk and resilience, multiculturalism, empowerment, and spirituality, and how they mesh with the recovery philosophy of mental illness.

The Value Base of Social Work Practice

All professions espouse distinct value bases that are intended to define their purposes and guide the actions of their members. Values are principles concerning what is right and good, while ethics are principles concerning what is right and correct; another way to describe ethics is as rules of conduct to which social workers should adhere (Dolgoff et al., 2009). People may adhere to several sets of values in their various life roles, which may be consistent with each other or in conflict. Personal values reflect one's own beliefs and preferences about what is right and good for oneself and others. Societal values reflect a consensus among members of a group about what is right and good that has been reached through negotiation, often politically. (Of course, there are differing social values with regard to the rights of persons with mental illness.)

Professional values guide the work of a person in his or her professional life. Professional ethics are the obligations of social workers in relationships with other people encountered in the course of their work, including consumers, other professionals, and the general public. Still, there are often conflicts among a social worker's personal, social, and professional values (which are open to interpretation), and these may create conflicts in the worker's efforts to work collaboratively with consumers.

The National Association of Social Workers (NASW) Code of Ethics (2008) is intended to serve as a guide to the professional conduct of social workers. The primary mission of the social work profession, according to the Code, is "to enhance human well-being and help meet the basic human needs of all people, with particular attention to the needs and empowerment of those who are vulnerable, oppressed, and living in poverty" (NASW, 2008, p. 1). The six core values of the profession, with their accompanying ethical principles, are

1. Service. Social workers' primary goal is to help people in need and to address social problems.
2. Social justice. Social workers challenge social injustice.
3. Dignity and worth of the person. Social workers respect the inherent dignity and worth of all people.
4. The importance of human relationships. Social workers recognize the central importance of human relationships in people's lives. (The Code goes on to assert that social workers engage people as partners in the helping process.)
5. Integrity. Social workers behave in a trustworthy manner.
6. Competence. Social workers practice within their areas of competence and develop and enhance their professional expertise.

In challenging social injustice, the Code of Ethics further states that social workers should "pursue social change, particularly with and on behalf of vulnerable and oppressed individuals and groups of people" (NASW, 2008, p. 6). Social workers should strive to ensure consumers' access to needed information, services, and resources, equality of opportunity, and meaningful participation in decision making. Social workers work with and on behalf of consumers as much as possible in a spirit of partnership. Thus, the value of social justice supports a social worker's collaborations with consumers, not only toward their personal fulfilment, but also in their battles against stigma and discrimination.

The major implication of the social worker's obligation to uphold professional values with regard to the selection of interventions is that the practitioner's activities should promote the mission of the profession. We will refer to these core values and how they are applied throughout the book, including how social workers may feel compelled to work against the wishes of consumers in some situations.

Strengths-Oriented Social Work Practice

Strengths-oriented practice implies that social workers should assess all consumers in light of their capacities, talents, competencies, possibilities, visions, values, and hopes (Saleebey, 2008). This perspective emphasizes human resilience, or the skills, abilities, knowledge, and insight that people accumulate over time as they struggle to surmount adversity and meet life challenges. It refers to the ability of consumers to persist in spite of their difficulties. In a recent research review it was found, for example, that when people are able to recognize or develop strengths after a major stressor, they experience less depression and a greater sense of well-being (Helgeson, Reynolds, & Tomich, 2006).

Dennis Saleebey (2008), the profession's foremost writer on this topic, asserts that many helping professionals have been historically guided by a deficits perspective, one that exists in opposition to humanistic values. This problem orientation encourages individual rather than social systems accounts of psychosocial functioning, which is contrary to social work's person-in-environment perspective. Saleeby notes several negative assumptions held by some professionals, including notions that the person is the problem (rather than person-in-environment interactions), that there are inevitable, critical, and universal stages of development, that childhood trauma invariably leads to adult psychopathology, and that there are certain social conditions so toxic that they invariably lead to problems in functioning for people, families, and groups.

The mental health professions' ongoing adherence to a deficits perspective is perpetuated by their cultural traditions, but it is also reinforced by managed care and insurance company reimbursement criteria that follow the medical model of assessment. Saleebey's work is constructive in offering positive concepts for social workers to use that can more readily identify consumer strengths. The major principles of strengths practice include the following:

- All people have strengths.
- Problems can be a source of both challenge and opportunity.
- Practitioners can never know the upper levels of consumers' growth potentials.
- There should be greater collaboration between practitioners and consumers to replace the traditional social worker–consumer hierarchy.
- Every environment includes resources (many of them informal) that can be mobilized to help consumers change.

One means by which a social worker can focus on consumer strengths is by paying attention to the following issues during the assessment process (Bertolino & O'Hanlon, 2002):

- Treatment history. What was helpful and not helpful in the past.
- Personal history. Physical, psychological, social, spiritual, and environmental assets. How the person has coped with stresses and challenges.
- Family history. Supportive relationships.
- Community involvement. Cultural and ethnic influences, community participation, spiritual and church involvement, neighborhood assets, other social supports.
- Employment and education. Achievements, skills, and interests.

By the time some consumers seek help from a social worker, their problems may have preoccupied them to an extent that they have lost sight of their resources. Indeed, Brun and Rapp (2001) identified in a qualitative study that an inability to initially accept the presence of strengths is a prominent theme among consumers with mental illness. When working from the strengths perspective, the social worker is alert to strengths and openly verbalizes them to consumers, but the consumer may only be likely to risk utilizing them if the relationship is strong.

A Risk and Protective Framework for Social Work Practice

The risk and protective framework considers the balance of mechanisms that interact to determine a consumer's ability to function adaptively despite stressful life events (Fraser, 2004). It provides a basis for social workers to identify and bolster consumer strengths and to reduce their risk influences.

- Risks are hazards in the individual or the environment that increase the likelihood of a problem occurring. The presence of a risk influence does not guarantee a negative developmental outcome, but it does increase the odds of one occurring.
- Protective influences involve the personal, social, and institutional resources that foster competence and promote successful development. They decrease the likelihood of the consumer engaging in problem behavior and increase the likelihood of a consumer rebounding from trauma and stress (Dekovic, 1999).
- Resilience refers to the absence of significant developmental delays and disabilities, or serious learning and behavior problems, and the mastery of developmental tasks that are appropriate for a person's age and culture, in spite of exposure to adversity (Werner & Altman, 2000).

Social work researchers have organized the risk and resilience framework into a biopsychosocial framework (Fraser, 2004). Relevant influences are considered with regard to a person's biological constitution, psychological status, and social environment. This framework fits well with social work's emphasis on empowerment and strengths. The strengths perspective underlies the concepts of protective influences and resilience in that people are not only able to endure, but also to triumph over difficult life circumstances, including those presented by serious mental illness.

The presence of a certain risk or protective influence may increase the likelihood of other such influences. For example, an aversive parenting style with poor monitoring increases the risk of children socializing with deviant peers (Smokowski, Mann, Reynolds, & Fraser, 2004). If parents are overwhelmed by environmental stresses such as unemployment, a lack of transportation and medical care, or living in an unsafe neighborhood, their ability to provide consistent nurturing may be compromised. This phenomenon also operates for protective influences. Adolescents whose parents provide emotional support and structure the environment with consistent rules and monitoring tend to associate with peers who share similar family backgrounds. Supportive parenting, in turn, affects the characteristics of the child in that he or she learns to regulate emotions and develop social competence. Social systems interactions also play themselves out from the basis of a child's characteristics. If a child has resilient qualities such as social skills, effective coping strategies, intelligence, and self-esteem, he or she is more likely to attract quality caregiving.

Although the exact nature of how risk and protective mechanisms work together is unknown, different mechanisms are hypothesized. Two primary models are the additive and the interactive models (Pollard, Hawkins, & Arthur, 1999). In an additive model, protective influences exert a positive effect to counterbalance the negative influences of risk. In an interactive model, protective influences enact a buffering function against risk. At times, risk and protective mechanisms are the converse of each other. For instance, at the individual level difficult temperament is a risk influence and easy temperament is a protective influence for problems in social functioning. Even though it is not easy to utilize knowledge of risk and protective mechanisms with specificity in assessment and intervention with persons who have mental illness, the social worker's attention to these balancing factors can sustain an orientation toward strengths and possibilities for consumer change.

Much remains to be learned about the specific risk and protective factors for most problems in living, and the ways in which these factors interact, but the framework encourages social workers to attend to these mechanisms in formulating individualized intervention plans. Social work's sensitivity to biological, psychological, and social risk and protective mechanisms is a professional value that can offer much to recovering consumers with mental illness. Such persons are engaged in a challenging, ongoing process of self-advancement by trying to understand and control their strengths and limitations, and the research knowledge being developed about these relative aspects of life can be helpful to that process. When consumers with mental illness talk about the challenges they face, social workers need to validate their full range of thoughts and feelings. They should always ask about the resilient qualities their consumers possess. As noted earlier, the social worker can inquire about aspects of the consumer's life that are intact despite the problem, and explore for resources they may draw upon in trying to cope with the problem. Questions can further center on personal or family qualities or strengths that have developed as a result of dealing with the presenting problem.

The Mail Sorter

Selma is a thirty-eight-year-old married Mexican American female with no children who lives in a rural county. She is court-ordered to attend a mental health clinic for anger management services. Selma has been diagnosed with bipolar I disorder, most recent episode mixed, with rapid cycling; and with alcohol abuse. Two months ago her husband charged her with assault after she stabbed him in the shoulder with a steak knife during an argument at a restaurant. She has been jailed on five occasions in her life for offenses ranging from disturbing the peace to assault. Following her arrests, she is typically released from jail after a few days into the custody of her husband, with the charges dropped.

Selma is in good physical health. She has kept a full-time job with the post office for the past fifteen years as a mail sorter and deliverer. She reports that she has had irritable and up and down moods most of her adult life. She describes extended periods when she becomes "hyperactive" and easily annoyed with people around her. Selma says she has "incredible energy" at those times and "gets a lot done." At those times, she likes delivering the mail, working out at the local recreation center, eating out at restaurants, and going to bars. She rests primarily with "short naps" during her energy bursts. Selma drinks beer regularly, and makes no apologies for it: "It's fun. Who says girls can't hold their liquor like the guys?" She says that she drinks only "enough to get drunk" when in a "high-energy" phase. Otherwise she limits herself to a few beers on the weekends.

Selma admits that she wears herself out after about a month of this hyperactivity, and becomes shaky and disoriented from a lack of sleep. When agitated, Selma becomes prone to losing her temper and argues with "almost anyone" who gets in her way. She gets into fights frequently, often with strangers, but sees this as acceptable behavior: "I was raised to take care of myself. No one is going to push me around." Despite her erratic behaviors, Selma is well known and "accepted for who I am" in her community. Her Mexican American culture features high levels of emotional expressiveness, and Selma is comfortable with this.

Selma says that she doesn't know why her energy bursts come and go. "I don't know, it's all about biorhythms, isn't it?" She admits to getting "really dark" for periods of time as well, sometimes for months at a time. She is barely able to get her work done at those times, admitting that her boss complains about her "laziness." When she is not in a "hyper" or "down" mood, as she says, Selma's moods tend to change throughout any given day. She is forgetful, easily distracted, cycling between not sleeping at all and sleeping too much, experiences bursts of energy and feelings of elation, decreased interest in her daily activities, feelings of sadness, and impulsive behavior.

When asked if it had ever been suggested that she had a mental problem, Selma sighs. "My doctor thinks I should take medicine for my moods, but I don't want to do that. I'm not a doper." Selma adds, "I'm usually pretty calm when I see my doctor. I don't go to him when I'm hyper." Selma does not recall that many people in her community have suggested professional intervention to her. "I can take care of myself. All of us had to learn to do that where I came from." Regarding her drinking, Selma does not exhibit signs of tolerance or withdrawal and has not increased her overall alcohol intake over the years.

Selma's mother was a homemaker who "stayed home most of the time and seemed sad. She never had any fun." She says her mother was nice but drank too much. Her father, a military veteran, was a "good man" who died when she was fourteen years old. She remembers always being an active child, but that she got "out of control" at about the time of her father's death. Her mother is still living, but moved to California with a second husband when Selma was twenty-two. They do not have a close relationship.

Selma has been married for fifteen years to a supportive husband. "He's a good man, a calm man, and he taught me to get more focused about my life." Carl, a manager at a local manufacturing plant, reports that he loves his wife. Selma and her husband both report financial difficulties that require her husband to work long hours, leaving Selma at home alone many evenings.

Selma has inconsistent contact with the people in the community. "I'm friendly with everyone, but nobody in particular." She was eager for her mandated treatment to end so that she could resume working. When asked about her possible sentencing to more time in jail, she shrugged. "I'm sorry for acting out like I do. I think the judge knows that. I'm a good person."

Risk and Protective Influences for Bipolar Disorder

Family history studies indicate a higher-than-average aggregation of bipolar disorder in families. Children with a bipolar parent have between a 2 and a 10 percent chance of developing the disorder (Youngstrom, Findling, Youngstrom, & Calabrese, 2005). Stressful life events may play an activating role in early episodes of bipolar disorder, with subsequent episodes arising more in the absence of clear external precipitants (Newman, 2006). Many of these life events are associated with social rhythm disturbances (sleep, wake, and activity cycles) (Berk et al., 2007). Persons with bipolar disorder who have a history of extreme early-life adversity, such as physical or sexual abuse, show an earlier age of onset, faster and more frequent cycling, increased suicidal ideation, and a presence of other problem conditions, including substance abuse (Post, Leverich, King, & Weiss, 2001).

Regarding its course, bipolar I disorder is highly recurrent, with 90 percent of persons who have a manic episode developing future episodes (Sierra, Livianos, Arques, Castello, & Rojo, 2007). The number of episodes tends to average four in ten years; approximately 50 percent of persons move through alternating manic and depressed cycles (Tyrer, 2006). About 10 percent experience rapid cycling (APA, 2000), which implies a poorer long-term outcome, since such persons are at a higher risk for both relapse and suicidal ideation. Women experience rapid cycling more than men do, possibly because of hormonal differences and natural changes in thyroid function (Barnes & Mitchell, 2005). A majority of those affected (70 to 90 percent) return to a stable mood and functioning capacity between episodes.

Persons with bipolar disorder tend to experience serious occupational and social problems (Marangell, Kupfer, Sachs, & Swann, 2006). One study indicated a stable working capacity in only 45 percent of clients, and a steady decline in job status and performance in 28 percent (Hirschfeld, Lewis, & Vornik, 2003). Missed work, poor work quality, and conflicts with coworkers all contribute to the downward trend for clients who cannot maintain mood stability. From 30 to 60 percent of persons with bipolar disorder fail to regain full function between episodes with regard to vocational and social performance.

Persons who experience high levels of life stress after the onset of bipolar disorder are four times more likely to have a relapse than are clients with low levels of life stress (Tyrer, 2006). One study found the relapse risk was related to both the lingering presence of symptoms of mania and to harsh comments from relatives (Schenkel, West, Harral, Patel, & Pavuluri, 2008).

Selma's Risk and Protective Influences

From a strengths perspective, a social worker would note that the presence of Selma's bipolar disorder was likely the result of an inherited biological condition. Selma's mother may have had a depressive disorder, given the client's description of her as "drinking too much" and being "sad" much of the time. If so, Selma would have had a higher-than-average risk of developing a mood disorder. Selma's risk influences for a poorer outcome of her bipolar condition include her rapid cycling, comorbid alcohol abuse, inconsistent structuring of her activities of daily life, and a lack of insight into the disorder, which has thus far resulted in her failure to seek help. She experiences protective influences as well, and the social worker would build on these in helping Selma recover from the cyclical nature of her problem. These include a relatively late age of onset (her early twenties), a stable and supportive husband, regular health check-ups, community support (with regard to her apparently sympathetic employer), and ongoing intervention (if she persists with the intervention). Additionally, Selma exudes a natural self-confidence that may contribute to her persistence in managing the disorder, if she commits to doing so.

Multiculturalism

All people with mental illnesses experience unique psychological and social challenges as they work toward optimal recovery. This is a basic tenet of the recovery philosophy, of course, but the process is further complicated by each person's membership in any of various racial and cultural groups, which influences how he or she views the world and his or her place in it. Persons from different cultures have different beliefs about the symptoms of mental illness, its causes, its consequences, its implications for social functioning, and appropriate ways of managing the symptoms; in some cultures, mental illnesses might not even be acknowledged as such. In order for social workers to understand consumers as best they can, it is imperative that they be sensitive to each consumer's cultural backgrounds.

Multiculturalism, or a social worker's ability to understand and work from the perspective of a variety of consumer cultures, represents an advance from the self-awareness that has always been a hallmark of the profession. The development of cultural competence is based on the principle that minority consumers—persons of racial and ethnic groups, gender, age, immigrant status, geographic background, sexual orientation, and disability that are different from the majority population—have their own ways of seeking and receiving assistance, and that these differences should be respected (Fong & Furuto, 2001).

Cultural competence demands an approach to consumers in which "assumptions are few and are held only until the truth becomes known" (Dorfman, 1996, p. 33). In Lee and Greene's (2003) model of social work education, two dimensions of competence, including cultural knowledge and cultural sensitivity, are the primary factors involved in providing effective transcultural intervention. Cultural knowledge refers to the practitioner's ability to acquire specific knowledge about his or her consumers' cultural background. Cultural sensitivity refers to a social worker's attitudes and values about cross-cultural direct practice.

Members of some cultures experience barriers to treatment due to providers' lack of awareness of cultural issues, biases, or inability to speak the consumer's language, as well as the consumer's mistrust of professional intervention (U.S. Department of Health & Human Services [DHHS], 2001). Social workers must realize that it is impossible to truly know cultures other than their own, but competent responses to transcultural helping situations should include high levels of both cultural knowledge and sensitivity. In addition to acquiring culture-specific knowledge about consumers, the competent practitioner must be able to maintain an informed and empathic response to them. When a social worker has developed a competent response to the transcultural helping situation, he or she can make judgments about intervention from an informed point of view, be open and sensitive in the cross-cultural helping situation, connect with consumers at an empathic level, and maintain awareness of his or her own personal experiences that might distort judgment.

It must be emphasized, however, that although multicultural competence has long been a value of many helping professions, it is more often discussed than evaluated. In their twenty-year content analysis of multicultural counseling competencies research, Worthington, Soth, and Moreno (2007) concluded that the literature consistently shows counselors who possess such competencies tend to evidence improved processes and outcomes with clients across racial and ethnic differences, but that there are methodological limitations associated with much of this literature. Those authors go on to say that there continues to be a need for new research on this topic that broadens the racial and ethnic composition of samples, uses real counselor–client dyads, and replicates existing findings across contexts and samples.

One example of a multicultural training program used for social workers and other behavioral health providers is Pennsylvania's Partners Reaching to Improve Multicultural Effectiveness (PRIME) (Stanhope et al., 2008). This is an eighteen-session, nine-month federal grant–funded program intended to transform provider attitudes, increase their knowledge, and enhance their skills for working with people who have mental health disabilities. Its effects were evaluated afterward with forty-two consumers who were surveyed about their perceptions of their providers' cultural competence. The consumers indicated that it was only moderately important to have a provider of the same cultural, racial, and ethnic group as themselves, and only moderately important that the provider address their cultural backgrounds in the service plan. These same consumers were moderately to very satisfied with their providers' inclusion of their cultural background into the intervention, and gave medium to high ratings of provider cultural competence. The researchers concluded that, while not all clients were overtly sensitive to their cultural issues being addressed, it was important to some of them to work at this level of specificity. More generally, most consumer respondents were satisfied with the apparent cultural competence of their providers who had completed the PRIME program.

Finally, it is sometimes assumed that a social worker working with a consumer who appears to be a member of his or her own culture is not a multicultural helping situation. Still, the similarities between a consumer and a social worker that appear on a surface may cloud awareness of their many possible differences, and this might disrupt the quality of the intervention process (Harper & Lantz, 2007). Surface characteristics are not always primary cultural indicators. Thus it is most constructive to assume that every practice situation is in reality a multicultural practice situation.

We now turn to a discussion of consumer empowerment in social work practice, a process by which consumers can be helped to utilize their existing strengths toward the achievement of goals in their recovery process.

Consumer Empowerment

In keeping with the profession's values and mission, social work practitioners at all levels desire to enhance the capacity, or power, of consumers to address their life concerns. Power can be understood as including

- A positive sense of self-worth and competence,
- The ability to influence the course of one's life,
- The capacity to work with others to control aspects of public life, and
- The ability to access the mechanisms of public decision making (Lee, 2001).

Many consumers do not, or perceive that they do not, have power, either over themselves, their significant others, or the agencies and communities in which they receive services and live. This sense of powerlessness can be internalized and lead to learned helplessness and alienation from one's community. These feelings may be intensified for persons dealing with mental illnesses, because they often face stigmatization and devaluing by others. An empowerment orientation to practice represents the social worker's efforts to combat the alienation, isolation, and poverty of substantive content in consumers' lives by promoting their sense of worth, sense of membership in a community, and ability to create change in their surroundings (Rose, 1990). "Don't go in with a mental blueprint of what empowerment looks like; it looks different for every individual" (Wallcraft, 1994, p. 8).

Empowerment incorporates three themes (Parsons, 1991). First, it is a developmental process that can be experienced along a continuum from individual growth to social change. Second, it is at least in part a psychological state characterized by feelings of self-esteem, efficacy, and control over one's life. The research has found that the concept of perceived control is related to a reduction in psychological stress and increased social action (Zimmerman, 2000). Third, it may involve a consumer's liberation from oppression, a process that begins with education and politicization of his or her problems with mental illness. Put another way, consumers may be empowered at a personal level (changing their patterns of thinking, feeling, and behaving), an interpersonal level (managing their relationships more effectively), or perhaps at a political level (changing their manner of interacting with larger systems) (Lee, 2001). Direct practice social workers are generally more inclined to address a consumer's personal and interpersonal levels. Empowerment at the individual level is a process by which consumers are helped to gain greater mastery and control over their lives, and a critical understanding of their environment (Zimmerman, 2000). In every case of empowerment practice, the social worker helps consumers with mental illness become aware of the conflicts and tensions within themselves and their surroundings that oppress or limit them, and helps them become better able to free themselves from those constraints. These constraints often pertain to the stigma and discrimination associated with mental disability.

One group of researchers has developed a goal instrument for quality procedure to help practitioners focus on empowerment themes when working with consumers in recovery (Clarke, Crowe, Oades, & Deane, 2009). This instrument, discussed more fully in the next chapter, urges practitioners to incorporate a recovery vision into any set of written goals with clients. Goals must be collaborative, include a scale indicating each one's relative importance to the consumer, and address the consumer's level of perceived self-efficacy in working toward each.

With their person-in-environment perspective on human functioning, social workers are well positioned to promote consumer empowerment. A key to empowerment practice is the social worker's awareness of the interactions between a consumer's problem situation and his or her capacity to interpret and act on the problem (Leonardson, 2007). For this process to be effective, social workers must possess knowledge about how organizations function, since they will be supporting consumer participation in various organizations; and they must be empowered themselves in ways that give them the competence to act with consumers. The sources of power over social workers in an agency (administrative or interprofessional) may create social worker–consumer power disparities that undermine the goals of empowerment practice. That is, if social workers have (or perceive that they have) limited influence in their own agencies, they will not be capable of empowering consumers in ways that may be at odds with the agency's own goals. For example, some agencies prohibit professional staff from participating in advocacy activities that place them in conflict with other community agencies, because this might place traditions of cooperation between these agencies at risk.

Social work practice is empowering to the extent that it helps people develop skills to become independent problem solvers and decision makers. The practitioner must be willing to teach consumers the knowledge and skills necessary to secure external resources and participate in social change activities if they so desire. Not all consumers seek interventions targeted toward all of these areas, but the social worker should have the capacity to initiate these change activities if so requested.

Empowerment Controversies

The capacity of the social work profession to further the interests of consumers has been a topic of concern among academic scholars (Ehrenreich, 1985). That is, while empowerment is a popular concept, it may be misunderstood, misused, and difficult to operationalize in practice in the following ways (Masterson & Owen, 2006):

- Professional power may be maintained by limiting the range of consumer decisions, and shaping consumer and professional roles to further an acceptance of expert authority.
- Professionals may resist what they consider to be unacceptable reconceptualizations of mental illness as promoted by some consumer groups.
- Professionals may disapprove of, and negatively influence, what they perceive to be radical advocacy activities by some consumers.

- Some practitioners may believe it is unethical to suggest goals and activities for consumers that do not directly relate to their presenting problems (Clark, 2000).
- Social workers may not be able to empower their consumers unless they themselves have more power (respect and influence) among their peers in the service professions.

All of these concerns will be addressed throughout this book.

The possible risks of the empowerment practice have been considered by other authors (Adams, 1996) and include the following:

- Some consumers prefer the social worker to be an expert, and wish to rely on his or her guidance in seeking solutions for their problems. They may be uncomfortable with empowerment practice.
- Empowerment may draw attention away from the immediate needs of the consumer. The person may not get his or her primary needs met if he or she, or the practitioner, shifts attention to macro-scale issues.
- The values on which empowerment is based may be conflicting. Self-determination, social justice, and democratic participation may be operationalized in ways that are in conflict with each other (Carroll, 1994). For example, one interest group's sense of self-determination (e.g., students with mental illness at a university who advocate for an expansion of formal disability services) may result in initiatives that attempt to usurp power from university administrators (e.g., who place student services priorities elsewhere). That is, empowerment is not necessarily a win-win proposition for members of different social groups.

The Mail Sorter Revisited

Selma, who was introduced earlier in this chapter, provides an example of a consumer who might prove to be an empowerment challenge for a social worker due to her frequent episodes of poor judgment. One immediate problem in this context is that she has been mandated to receive mental health services. Given her situation, the social worker might try to empower Selma at the individual and interpersonal levels, helping her to develop a better sense of competence and an ability to influence the course of her life toward her personal goals. One way to proceed would be for the social worker to help Selma identify her short- and long-term goals and then consider what behaviors would most likely help her achieve them. Selma would probably agree that she wants to avoid further legal and marital trouble, and the social worker might suggest that she could achieve this goal by learning to manage her moods and outbursts more effectively. So far, so good. Still, Selma might object to the intervention strategies of learning about her illness (which she denies having), taking medications (which is considered important to controlling bipolar disorder), drinking less, and maintaining a stricter lifestyle routine. The social worker might frame these interventions as facilitating Selma's potential to develop more effective personal power in her life, but the consumer might see them as dehumanizing, and refuse them. Selma might want the social worker to help her advocate with the legal system for fairer treatment, or support what she perceives as her assertive feminism in how she deals with interpersonal conflicts.

To summarize, empowerment is a concept that is useful for guiding social work practice at all levels. Despite its limitations, it has the potential to help consumer groups develop more secure lives through substantive interpersonal and community connections. The actions of social workers can always be productively driven by a concern with consumers' capacities to take control of their own lives.

Empowerment and Research

We saw in the last chapter that many consumers are skeptical about EBP research because it often involves large-scale quantitative research that may treat consumers as diagnostic types rather than as unique individuals. Intervention research from the empowerment perspective is conducted differently from traditional methods in which the professional is the expert and in control of the process. Empowerment research involves doing with rather than doing to, and emphasizes social worker–consumer collaboration (Boog, Coenen, & Keune, 2001). Intervention research uses consumers as participants rather than subjects in the areas of research design, accountability, implementation, and utilization. An example of empowerment research might be a social worker's meeting with members of a consumer drop-in center to discuss possible ways of evaluating the center's effectiveness. Members would be invited to participate in the design of the project, data-gathering activities, and decisions about how the results are used. More effort would be put into hearing and recording the perspectives of individuals about the services they receive.

Such research can also be used to assess how comfortable social workers are with facilitating consumer empowerment processes; several qualitative studies illustrate this point. In a study of twenty-eight consumers and social workers (including administrators) in a community-based service setting, frontline workers were interviewed about their perceptions of the empowerment process (Everett, Homstead, & Drisko, 2007). The researchers found that social workers sometimes experienced role conflicts in the process of helping consumers become more involved in their own problem-solving activities, moving back and forth from the roles of expert authority, to collaborator, to outreach worker. These workers were often challenged by the apparent powerlessness of their consumers to make changes in their lives, and felt the same sense of powerlessness at times in dealing with organizational barriers and limits in the scope of their job roles. Everett and colleagues concluded that for empowerment practice to be effective, the process must be supported at all levels of an organization. In another study of 145 consumers and professionals, Boehm and Staples found that the two parties sometimes had different perspectives on empowerment practice (Boehm & Staples, 2002). Consumers were more interested in the practical, tangible outcomes of empowerment activities, while social workers were more interested in the broad process of empowering consumers, with less of a focus on specific outcomes.

The difficulty of implementing empowerment-based practice was demonstrated in another qualitative study of practitioner perceptions of empowerment (Ackerson & Harrison, 2000). The eight practitioners in this study, who worked with highly impaired consumers at a mental health clinic, noted empowerment dilemmas related to the practical limits of their roles in practice, issues of control in the clinical relationship, and interprofessional conflicts. The practitioners believed that empowerment was a sometimes impractical goal; they perceived a need to exert control over consumers at times when the person's judgment appeared to be poor or their behavior dangerous. Balancing occasional directives with empowerment values was difficult for them. The participants also noted that it was difficult for them to support consumer empowerment activities among other members of a treatment team who did not observe this value. For example, the social workers supporting a consumer's active participation in considering what medications he or she should take may be met with strong resistance by a prescribing physician who does not support that level of consumer involvement. Ackerson and Harrison concluded that many social workers seem to define empowerment at a personal level that does not capture the breadth of the concept, and that there is tension between promoting consumer self-direction and acting on the consumer's behalf. The practitioners in this study did reach consensus on one component of empowerment: there should always be mutually agreed on roles in which the consumer and social worker share some responsibility and power.

While the above discussion may seem discouraging to social workers and consumers who value empowerment, it does illustrate the challenges in promoting empowerment in the current service world, where the medical model of care remains powerful.

Spirituality in Recovery Practice

The term "spirituality" has many definitions, but can be generally understood as a person's search for and adherence to meanings, purposes, and commitments that lie outside the self (adapted from Krill, 1996). Meaning-in-life issues are central to the recovery process, and social work's attention to these aspects of consumers' lives is critical. There are two contrasting perspectives on spirituality (Frankl, 1988). One is that people may create what is meaningful in their lives. That is, there are no objective or external sources of meaning that people must observe. Meanings emerge within people and reflect their interests and values. An example is the person who chooses to devote her life to working with abused children, having realized that doing so fulfils a personal preference that is also important to society. The second perspective holds that at least some meanings reflect a reality that exists independently of individuals. It becomes each person's challenge to discover meanings that exist objectively. Some religious groups believe that there is a divine plan and a correct set of beliefs about a Supreme Being and codes of conduct, and that persons should live in accordance with this plan. It is possible to hold both views simultaneously. That is, people may consider some purposes to be universal and others to be based on their individual searches for meaning.

When working with consumers around their orientations to spirituality and religion, it is important for social workers to understand the distinction between the two concepts (Russinova & Cash, 2007). Spirituality tends to be identified primarily with an individual's experience of the transcendent, whereas religion tends to be associated with institutional representations of the divine. Spiritual concerns are informal, personal, intrinsic, exploratory, and evolving, whereas religion is more organized, communal, extrinsic, prescriptive, and ritualistic. These ideas, which are a key part of one's recovery process, will be more fully addressed in chapter 6.

Summary

The reality of mental health practice today, across professional groups, is that consumers are usually offered a limited range of formal services and have limited opportunities to participate in making these choices. In contrast, a key point of the recovery philosophy is that it is not the role of social workers to make all decisions for consumers. Consumer-centered empowerment practice is highly consistent with the mission of the social work profession.

Consumers should be included from the beginning in decisions regarding their care. When consumers decide that they want to do something, their decisions ought to be respected, and the social workers should make reasonable efforts to assist. This is not to suggest, however, in programs such as drop-in centers, that consumer choice should be supported to the detriment of other consumers or program rules. Program rules that are set for the benefit of all should not have exceptions made in the name of the recovery philosophy. Consumers who do not agree with the rules of a particular program have the right to find a program that will better suit their needs.

Furthermore, if a consumer makes a decision that is contrary to the social worker's judgment, then the practitioner needs to help the consumer understand any reservations. A social worker may, for example, become concerned that a consumer's decision is likely to cause harm to him- or herself, or to someone else. Social workers have a responsibility articulated in the Code of Ethics to intervene "to prevent serious, foreseeable, and imminent harm to a consumer or other identifiable person" (NASW, 2008, p. 7). When a consumer's decision is not likely to cause serious harm, but still seems to the social worker to indicate poor judgment, the professional's responsibility is to educate the consumer about the possible consequences of that decision, but in the end let the consumer make those decisions.

In summary, social workers have an obligation to serve, support, and encourage consumers to do what their professional experience tells them is best. They must understand and accept that helping consumers to make their own choices will ultimately be in the best interests of their recovery, even if the social worker believes that some actions may have adverse consequences for the consumer. The recovery philosophy does not call for social workers to support activities they believe are unrealistic, would hinder the recovery of other consumers, or would involve treating one consumer more favorably than another. The philosophy calls for social workers to support consumers' decisions, within reason, to the best of their abilities, however.

Major Chapter Learning Points

- The value base of the social work profession supports collaboration with consumers toward their personal fulfilment and is consistent with the values of the recovery philosophy.
- Social work's sensitivity to consumers' strengths, along with attention to their biological, psychological, and social risk and protective mechanisms, potentiates consumers' development of realistic recovery goals.
- For social workers to fully understand consumers and their strivings, it is imperative that they possess cultural knowledge and cultural sensitivity.
- Empowerment is a process by which social workers help consumers take greater control of and responsibility for their recovery processes. Social work practice is empowering when it helps people develop skills to become more-independent problem solvers.
- Consumers may be empowered at personal, interpersonal, and political levels.
- Spiritual or meaning-in-life issues are central to the recovery process as consumers strive to make sense of their ongoing growth and adaptive challenges.

Questions for Reflection or Discussion

1. Think about one or two practice situations in which your personal values might conflict with any of social work's professional values. How might you resolve these dilemmas in working with a hypothetical consumer?

2. It was noted that consumers are often unable to perceive their strengths, even as the social worker identifies them. How can a social worker help a consumer own a strength, and risk utilizing it? Furthermore, to what extent should a social worker articulate a consumer's major limitations?

3. Consider one or two types of diverse client groups (age, race, ethnicity, gender, sexual orientation, socioeconomic status) about which you have little knowledge. What are three ways that you could develop cultural competence for working with these persons?

4. Think about one specific dilemma related to your own sense of responsibility or socially sanctioned power you might face in working with a consumer who wishes to assume control over some aspect of his or her life. Can you still be empowering in this situation?

Chapter 4

A Social Work Model of Recovery Practice (and Some Others)

A practice model, in contrast to a practice philosophy, is a concrete guiding strategy for human services professionals to follow in providing, in this case, recovery-oriented services to consumers; or for consumers to follow in their own recovery processes. A case was made in chapter 3 that the social work profession is well suited to adopt the recovery philosophy in its practices with such consumers. In this chapter, a flexible model of recovery practice for social workers will be described in some detail, and two subsequent chapters will elaborate on implications of that model. Prior to presenting the social work model, however, it will be useful to review some recovery models that have been developed by administrators, professionals, and consumer groups. These will familiarize the reader with initiatives already under way in the domain of recovery practice.

Recovery at the Systems Level

The resources available to social workers and their consumers, as determined by administrative priorities, affect the scope of interventions they may undertake together. Social workers, in fact, have a responsibility to participate in, and advocate for, agency, community, state, and even federal initiatives that may facilitate the development of recovery services for consumers.

The New Freedom Commission on Mental Health, described in chapter 2, endorsed the recovery philosophy as a basis for service provision for persons with mental illness; that vision has been adopted by mental health administrators in other countries as well as in the United States. Canadian researchers, for example, have argued that a recovery system of care implies five changes to existing services: more egalitarian relationships between service providers and users, a reorientation of support systems in keeping with consumers' own goals, a broadening of system supports to encompass life meaning issues, the provision of leadership roles for consumers, and the promotion of consumer-led services (Latimer, Bond, & Drake, 2011). A review of recovery systems implications in Australia, England, and New Zealand noted the five themes of service restructuring, promoting mental health as a holistic concept, developing a recovery-minded workforce, cultivating consumer partnerships, and establishing measurable outcome-oriented intervention practices (Piat & Sabetti, 2009).

The range of micro (direct practice) and macro (policy) recovery needs that consumers may experience has been outlined by Liberman (2008) and Davidson, Harding, et al. (2006). These include, with implications for the micro practice level, traditional employment, psychosocial rehabilitation, case management, therapy or counseling, advocacy assistance, self-help service opportunities, consumer and family psychoeducation, family-aided assertive community treatment (ACT), and dual disorders programs. At the macro level, recovery initiatives may address consumer needs in such areas as citizenship rights, setting system level program standards, and methods for planning and evaluating community-based mental health systems. What follows is one example of how these directives are addressed at a state level.

A State Model of Recovery Service Organization

The New Freedom Commission did not attach additional federal funding for implementing its vision, but its report mobilized mental health advocacy groups and spurred many state departments to incorporate this vision (Mechanic, 2008). As one example, the policies of the Ohio Department of Mental Health (ODMH, 2011) illustrate the potential of the states to assume leadership in promoting the recovery philosophy. (Ohio is the author's home state and is considered a national leader in the promotion of recovery services.) The state has articulated a desire to enhance recovery supports for consumers in the areas of employment, cultural competence of providers, housing, stigma reduction, faith-based initiatives, and consumer–family partnerships. In its mission statement, ODMH (2011) has articulated a commitment to the following principles:

- People can and do recover from mental illness.
- Nurturing resiliency helps children, youth, and families to successfully meet life's challenges.
- Services are most effective when delivered in culturally competent ways.
- Consumer and family involvement in the planning, evaluation, and delivery of services is vital.
- A focus on quality and continuous improvement is key to achieving an effective, person-centered mental health system.

To operationalize these principles, Ohio has established an Office of Consumer Recovery and Supports for the purpose of collaborating with consumers, families, boards, agencies, advocacy groups, state and national organizations, and other ODMH offices toward an implementation of the recovery vision.

The New Freedom Commission has been criticized for not specifying organizational changes that might bring existing service systems together. Still, all states are required to devote a portion of their block grant monies to recovery services. The following example is provided to show how implementation has been addressed by one direct practice agency.

The Harrison County Community Services Board

The Harrison County Community Services Board (CSB) is one of Ohio's forty comprehensive public mental health organizations. Renae Sands, Harrison County's Coordinator of Adult and Mental Health Services (personal communication, 2011), described the recovery systems transformation that is taking place at the Harrison CSB and other similar agencies across the state. The systems' transformation got under way in 2005 when policies were enacted at the state level, with modest funding attached, to include consumers at all levels of agency operations. During these past eight years, the CSB administrators have focused much of their attention on implementing recovery-oriented practices. These include the staff's use of recovery-focused language, becoming more consumer centered in service delivery, and providing recovery-focused assessments. There is now a clear differentiation between professional treatment and consumer self-help in some programs.

One of the CSB's first actions was to put together a recovery task force, consisting of five staff and five consumers, to examine the degree to which agency services were meeting the needs of consumers. The first activity it developed was a process for educating each sector (consumers and staff) about their unique perspectives on the intervention process. That is, consumers needed to better understand staff functions and perspectives, and vice versa. The administrative staff at the Harrison CSB discovered that consumers are quite assertive at the agency, which staff considers to be a good thing. Consumers are vocal about what they do and don't like. Agency administrators hope that this is an indicator of a collaborative atmosphere and mutual respect.

Another prominent way the CSB has engaged with its consumers is through an ongoing recovery-oriented outcome study. All consumers are periodically invited to complete the Recovery-Oriented Systems Inquiry (ROSI), a forty-two-item, five-point Likert survey that serves to evaluate the agency in the domains of service access, appropriateness, and quality, and a variety of outcomes formulated from the consumer perspective (National Association of State Mental Health Program Directors, 2012). Staff also conduct semiannual focus groups with consumers to flesh out the findings of these surveys. The collection of these data is mandated by, and later forwarded to, the state for incorporation with its own recovery research.

Like many agencies of its type, the Harrison CSB provides services to consumers with serious mental illnesses through intensive community treatment (ICT) teams that include approximately fifty consumers each. Each team comprises a nurse, five case managers (one of whom serves as a lead clinician), a peer specialist (a consumer), and a supervisor. Each team has access to one of the two part-time agency psychiatrists who perform medication evaluations. The agency also provides other services with a recovery focus. For example, it employs an adult outpatient team that focuses on work with persons who have substance abuse problems, a children's in-home team, and a crisis (emergency services) team.

The ICT reserves one staff position for a consumer, in keeping with the state's recovery and peer-run service ideals. An abbreviated job description for that person reads as follows:

> The incumbent is responsible for assisting agency staff to provide mental health supports to consumers who reside independently or in a supervised facility in the community. Provides training and support to enable consumers to achieve and maintain community stability and independence in the most

appropriate and least restrictive environment. Activities and services include training/teaching of supported living skills, activities of daily living, orientation to client's environment, nutrition, assistance with medication management, and other activities related to the consumers' mental and physical health. Adheres to all policies, procedures, regulations, documentation standards, and confidentiality requirements.

Essential tasks include intensive outreach and support at their residences and in the community. Assists consumers in understanding illness, symptoms identification, and coping skills. Teaches social skills, proper hygiene, and conflict resolution. Meets with primary case managers to provide feedback regarding problems. Attends staff meetings, weekly supervision, and in-service training as available. Assists consumers in accessing natural community supports. Arranges transportation to medical/clinical appointments and other community activities. Teaches and helps practice use of public transportation.

The peer specialist provides a full range of recovery services to consumers, including assessment, supportive counseling, medication support, and community integration. Additionally, unique roles of the peer specialist include taking consumers on casual outings for rapport building, leading Wellness Recovery Action Plan (WRAP) groups (to be discussed later in this chapter), and helping consumers formulate and carry out their WRAP plans. On the other hand, because of limited credentials, the peer specialist does not have primary responsibility for managing a caseload or for service documentation. Neither does the staff member conduct crisis or prescreening assessments for possible involuntary hospitalization, or participate in the team's twenty-four-hour coverage rotation. Still, this person is a full-time, paid member of the ICT, with the stipulation that he or she receive mental health services at a different agency. A second peer specialist is employed at the agency's consumer clubhouse. These persons receive lower salaries than other ICT staff because of their lower levels of training and preparation. This may change to some degree, however, because peer specialists can now receive certification by completing a regionally developed training program.

The concept of the peer specialist on treatment teams was developed by psychiatric rehabilitation professionals in Boston (Liberman, 2008). A literature review (including eight randomized control studies) examining the outcomes of having consumer providers on case management teams concluded that findings are mixed (Wright-Berryman, McGuire, & Salyers, 2011). That is, there was evidence supporting peer services for improving consumer engagement and limited support for reduced hospitalizations. Evidence was lacking, however, for other outcomes such as symptom reduction or improved quality of life. More-rigorous research is needed to further evaluate the impact of having consumer providers on teams.

Professional Models of Recovery

Several examples of recovery programs that exist at the micro, or direct-practice, level follow. These are not representative of the range of programs available, but illustrate how recovery practices can be implemented. First three models developed by professionals, and then three examples of consumer-developed recovery models are presented.

Collaborative Recovery Model   The Collaborative Recovery Model (CRM), which originated in Australia, provides an example of a semi-structured intervention for use with consumers who have mental illness (Marshall, Oades, & Crowe, 2009; Oades et al., 2005). Its guiding principles are that recovery is an individual process, and one that always emphasizes hope, a process of redefining identity, finding meaning in life, and taking responsibility for recovery; and that services must focus on social worker–consumer collaboration and the support of consumer autonomy, which involves intervention choices. The authors of CRM argue that their model provides an integrative framework combining EBP, competencies relevant to case management and psychosocial rehabilitation, and recognition of the subjective experiences of consumers. Practitioners who wish to utilize the CRM receive two full days of training in the model, followed by booster sessions six and twelve months later. The four semistructured components of CRM are the following:

1. Change enhancement. A process of engagement in which the practitioner addresses consumers' motivational and cognitive capacities by helping them identify change areas about which they feel ambivalent or energized.
2. Collaborative needs identification, using formal measures.
3. Collaborative goal setting and striving (using measures with a focus on both promoting change and preventing the occurrence of future problems). This includes a balancing of the importance of each goal to the consumer with its perceived manageability, using both proximal (short-term) and distal (long-term) goals, attending to the consumer's recovery vision, and utilizing three-

month incremental goals that facilitate ongoing service evaluation. (The details of proximal and distal goals will be described later in the chapter.)

4. Collaborative task assignment and monitoring, involving homework administration and a range of strategies for identifying and overcoming obstacles to completing the assignments.

In a quasi-experimental study to evaluate the impact of CRM, researchers focused on the experiences of consumers engaged in recovery support practices as well as their valuing of these activities (Marshall et al., 2009). Ninety-two adult consumers from metropolitan, regional, and rural mental health services in eastern Australian states were included in the study. It was found that consumers using services provided by CRM-trained workers identified significant changes to service delivery in relation to the frequency with which they were encouraged to take responsibility for their recovery, the degree to which they collaborated with staff, and the extent to which they were encouraged to complete homework activities to assist them in goal achievement, when compared with those using traditional services. The key aspects of CRM were valued by consumers, but no differences were found between the two groups in terms of ratings of practitioner helpfulness in assisting their recovery.

Across Boundaries   Across Boundaries (2012) is a mental health center in Toronto, unique in that it provides support services to people of color who experience mental illnesses. The organization operates under a holistic, recovery-oriented service philosophy and further utilizes an active, antioppression framework. With a staff of approximately twenty-two persons, including sixteen case managers and one consumer initiative coordinator, Across Boundaries is a registered charitable organization funded by Canada's Ministry of Health and Long-Term Care. In addition to providing direct services, the center also provides consultations and trainings to other agencies in the area.

Across Boundaries recognizes the interdependence of physical, mental, emotional, social, and spiritual factors in a person's life, but it focuses equal attention on economic, cultural, linguistic, and other environmental influences. Consumer services integrate skill building, social and recreational activities, individual and group support, alternative and complementary therapies, art therapies, a community kitchen, and community outreach. Most services are offered in-house, with the exceptions of some case management, family support, and outreach programs. Across Boundaries is committed to community development and to the active participation of communities of color. It recognizes that individual or systemic racism and oppression affects the health and mental health of minority persons and communities, and is a barrier to their accessing such services. It also recognizes diversity among racialized people who may face discrimination based on religion, language, ethnicity, class, gender, sexual orientation, disability, age, country of origin, and citizenship status. Its antioppression work focuses in part on providing opportunities for service providers to achieve cultural competence.

Antioppressive practice is a significant focus of mental health intervention in many agencies in Canada and is worthy of elaboration. This practice can be defined as a commitment to social justice that includes a clear theoretical and value base promoting egalitarianism, an understanding of one's social location and how it informs relationships and practice behaviors, a challenge to existing social relationships in which powerful groups maintain influence over less-powerful groups, and specific practice behaviors that minimize power imbalances and promote equity and empowerment for consumers (Larson, 2008). Specifically related to recovery work, establishing "just" working relationships under this definition includes

- Avoiding the use of titles, positions, and qualifications,
- Not using judgments in the form of diagnostic categories,
- Using appropriate self-disclosure,
- Providing and explaining all relevant information to consumers to demystify practice,
- Inviting consumers to participate in all decisions regarding their care,
- Assuring consumers they have the right to ask questions and to feel as they choose, and
- Providing a user-friendly environment for interviews and sessions.

Clearly, Across Boundaries incorporates the value that social workers and consumers should have egalitariam relationships, and its emphasis in this way goes beyond what many other recovery programs maintain.

The Illness Management and Recovery Model   The Illness Management and Recovery (IMR) model (Roe, Hasson-Ohayon, Salyers, & Kravetz, 2009) is a curriculum-based intervention for helping consumers acquire the knowledge and skills needed to manage their illnesses effectively and to achieve their recovery goals. IMR was developed as part of a National Implementing Evidence Based Practices Project, with input from a committee including researchers, practitioners, consumers, family members, and social service program leaders. It is based on the Transtheoretical Model of Change (TMOC), in which a consumer's ambivalence about addressing certain problems is first identified and then processed; and on a stress-vulnerability model of coping, which targets both a consumer's biological predisposition to the symptoms of mental illness, and the role of social support in reducing its risk. The developers of the IMR assert the program is unique because it includes emphases on goal setting, education, skills training, and motivational interventions.

It is worth describing the TMOC in some detail here because it is also utilized in the first component of the CRM. The TMOC provides a conceptualization of the general change process that all people go through when they are considering, or being asked to consider, making a significant behavioral change (Prochaska & DiClemente, 1982). It recognizes that people are often ambivalent about making changes in their lives, and their ambivalence needs to be openly addressed by a practitioner in order to help them resolve it in one direction or another. The five steps involved in the TMOC change framework are (1) precontemplation (denying the exisence of a problem behavior), (2) contemplation (considering the pros and cons of change), (3) preparation (planning for change), (4) action, and (5) maintenance. Ambivalence may persist through all five stages, although it is most prominent in the first three.

The IMR model also emphasizes the importance of setting both proximal and distal goals. Proximal (short-term and concrete) goals help consumers learn the fundamentals of illness self-management based on the stress-vulnerability model. Distal (longer-term and more abstract) goals help clients make progress toward recovery by addressing both objective (community functioning, social relationships, work) and subjective (sense of purpose, hope, confidence) dimensions of recovery. IMR practitioners draw from five empirically supported intervention

strategies: psychoeducation, cognitive-behavioral approaches to medication adherence, relapse prevention, social skills training, and coping
skills training. The IMR model addresses the following nine topics over
a series of ten program modules:

1. Recovery strategies
2. Practical facts about schizophrenia
3. The stress-vulnerability model and its related treatment strategies
4. Building social support
5. Using medications effectively
6. Reducing the frequency of relapses
7. Coping with stress
8. Coping with problems and persistent symptoms
9. Getting one's needs met in the mental health system

Either individual or group sessions can be provided, depending on the
nature of the agency and its consumer population; sessions are held
weekly for ten months, with the consumers' significant others involved
when possible. Providers utilize a variety of intervention tools and
strategies, including handouts, interactive teaching, reviews of information, regularly checking for consumer understanding, motivational
techniques to help consumers find reasons to change behavior and
develop hope for their futures, cognitive restructuring, and behavior
interventions, including positive reinforcement, shaping, modeling, role
playing, and relaxation training.

The standard structure of each IMR session includes informal
socializing with groups, a review of content covered during the previous
sessions, a review of homework assignments, follow-up discussions on
the status of consumer goals, setting agendas for the current session,
teaching new material and practicing new strategies, collaboratively formulating homework assignments for the next week, and summarizing
progress made in the current session.

The IMR model has been evaluated rather extensively. Salyers,
Godfrey, et al. (2009) evaluated the statewide implementation of the program in Indiana. The Assertive Community Treatment Center of Indiana
assisted seven community mental health centers with implementation of
the program. At six and twelve months, the fidelity of its implementation
was assessed, and changes in illness self-management, hope, and satisfaction with services were assessed for 324 consumers. It was found that the

IMR program was successfully implemented at six of seven sites. The self-reports of consumers and practitioners indicated significant changes in illness self-management at those sites. Consumers also reported increased hope, but no changes in satisfaction with their services.

Salyers, Hicks, and McGuire (2009) conducted an uncontrolled, nine-month pilot study to determine whether a peer specialist could be effectively trained to provide IMR on an established ACT team. This study included both quantitative measures of knowledge and recovery beliefs, and qualitative interviews with fourteen consumers and sixteen providers. Results indicated that consumer perceptions of recovery significantly improved with the addition of the IMR model, and that there was a trend toward their increased knowledge. Both consumers and staff reported many benefits of IMR, including an increase in consumers' willingness to try new things and be involved in more meaningful activities, and greater hope for both consumers and staff. The integration of IMR onto ACT with a peer specialist thus shows promise as a way to improve consumer recovery outcomes and increase the recovery orientation of ACT.

An earlier study described the development and theoretical underpinnings of the IMR program and presented data from the United States and Australia, using twenty-four consumers who had either schizophrenia or schizoaffective disorder, on the effects of individual-based and group-based IMR treatment over the nine-month program and three-month follow-up periods (Mueser et al., 2006). Most participants reported high levels of satisfaction. Furthermore, strong improvements during treatment and at follow-up were found in clients' effectiveness in coping with their symptoms and clinicians' reports of their global functioning, with moderate improvements in consumer knowledge about mental illness, symptom-related distress, hope, and goal orientation. A later study considered the longer-term impact of IMR (Roe et al., 2009). Thirty-six people with serious mental illness were interviewed one year after completing IMR, and a qualitative analysis of their responses revealed high levels of perceived program helpfulness. Domains of improvement included cognition, coping, and social support.

Another group of resarchers evaluated the effectiveness of the IMR model provided in a group format. A total of 210 persons with severe mental illness receiving treatment at rehabilitation centers in a community in Israel were randomly assigned to either the IMR program or treatment as usual. Participants in IMR demonstrated significant improvement in knowledge about their illness and progress toward their personal goals, compared with those receiving treatment as usual. Clinician ratings also indicated significant improvement in overall outcome for IMR clients compared with those who received treatment as usual. Significant improvement in coping was found in both groups, and no differences were found in either group in the area of social support.

Three examples of consumer-generated recovery programs are presented next.

Recovery Models Developed By Consumers

Wellness Recovery Action Plan   The Wellness Recovery Action Plan (WRAP) is a structured system for consumer self-care developed in the late 1980s by Mary Ellen Copeland (2008). It offers a systematic way for consumers to reduce the severity and frequency of their symptoms of mental illness. WRAP is offered as a psychoeducational program by trained consumers in group settings, and incorporates the goals of promoting personal, organizational, and community wellness. After a consumer has developed a personalized WRAP plan, he or she can continuously review and update the plan with the assistance of a WRAP provider or peer specialist. The Copeland Center for Wellness and Recovery (http://copelandcenter.com/) is the only organization that provides the training required for the consumer to become a certified WRAP facilitator.

WRAP incorporates the five key principles of hope, personal responsibility, education, self-advocacy, and support, and works to shift the focus in mental health care from control of symptoms to recovery. WRAP participants are encouraged to take responsibility for their own wellness by using a variety of self-help techniques provided in a workbook and reaching out for assistance to their network of family, friends, and health-care providers. The intended outcomes of a consumer's WRAP involvement are life enhancement and gains in self-esteem and self-confidence, and becoming a more fully contributing member of the community. The same topics are covered in each WRAP program, but they are tailored to individual sets of participants. Topics include improving self-esteem; changing negative thoughts to positive ones; developing peer support; addressing work-related issues; recovering from trauma; preventing suicide; and securing appropriate living space, lifestyle, and motivation. Courses may be offered through consumer organizations, but WRAP is also offered as a part of the programming of many social services agencies.

Through the time-limited group intervention (these can be variable, but often feature two-hour weekly sessions for eight weeks), WRAP promotes each consumer's development of a wellness toolbox, or a list of resources he or she can utilize to stay healthy and deal with challenges. The WRAP workbook includes many individualized strategies for achieving goals. A consumer's WRAP plan consists of six parts:

1. The daily maintenance plan: A description of the well self and lists of things one must do to maintain wellness
2. Triggers: Things outside the self that can happen to make one feel worse
3. Early warning signs: Subtle signs that let the person know he or she may soon feel worse
4. When things are breaking down: Signs that the person is feeling much worse and in danger of experiencing a crisis, with tools for how to constructively respond
5. Crisis planning and advance directives: Identification of symptoms for sharing with significant others that indicate they should take over responsibility for the consumer's care and decision making, health-care information, as well as a plan for staying at home and receiving appropriate support
6. Postcrisis planning: Guidelines enabling the person to gradually resume life as it was before the crisis

WRAP has proven to be a popular consumer-led program nationally and has been evaluated numerous times. One recent quasi-experimental study with 114 participants examined the effects of WRAP participation on consumers' symptoms, hope, and recovery outcomes (Fukui et al., 2011). Eight- to twelve-week WRAP sessions were facilitated by one staff person and one peer worker at five community mental health centers in a Midwestern state. Change measures were completed at the first and last WRAP sessions, as well as at six months after the intervention. Findings revealed significant group intervention effects for the variables of symptoms and hope, but not for recovery markers. Group comparisons showed significant improvements for the experimental group with regard to psychiatric symptoms and hope after the intervention, and nonsignificant changes for the comparison group. In another study, researchers assessed three dimensions of self-management (attitudes, knowledge, and skills) among consumers participating in WRAP programs representing statewide initiatives in Vermont and Minnesota (Cook et al., 2010). Pre- and postcomparisons were made of reports from 381 participants (147 in Vermont and 234 in Minnesota) on various outome measures. Significant positive changes were observed in all three dimensions on 76 percent (thirteen of seventeen) of items completed by Vermont participants, and 85 percent (eleven of thirteen) of items completed by Minnesota participants. In both states, participants reported significant increases in hopefulness for their recovery, awareness of their early warning signs of decompensation, the use of wellness tools in their daily routines, awareness of symptom triggers, having a crisis plan, having a plan for dealing with symptoms, having a social support system, and perceiving the ability to take responsibility for their own wellness.

The Virginia Organization of Consumers Advocating Leadership   The Virginia Organization of Consumers Advocating Leadership (VOCAL) is a statewide consumer-run organization of 1,300 members that seeks to strengthen the formal mental health services system by creating alternatives and complements to it. Through its offices in two cities, VOCAL works to educate people with mental health challenges about how to become and stay well, and it keeps consumers connected so they can strengthen one another through mutual actions of self-determination and peer leadership. Run by a fourteen-member board of directors, a paid executive director, and seven other paid, part-time staff, VOCAL operates with the following guiding values:

- We value and work for the full human rights and self-determination of every individual, regardless of his or her mental state or diagnosis.
- We encourage individual input into creating a truly healing mental-health-care system.
- We value each person's individual process of mental health recovery.
- We value the worth and dignity of all people.

Partial funding for VOCAL comes from the state's mental health block grant, and additional funds are acquired from sponsorships and grants. The organization's activities are directed in the areas of advocacy, community building, recovery education, and grassroots programming. VOCAL is responsible for four major programs, including Recovery Education and Creative Healing (REACH), the VOCAL Consumer Owned and Operated Programs (CO-OP; a collection of peer-run mental health programs), the VOCAL Network (a statewide network of people in recovery), and the dissemination of a book, *Firewalkers*. Each of these programs is described below.

Recovery Education and Creative Healing   The purpose of the Recovery Education and Creative Healing (REACH) is to advance the principles of recovery through consumer education and training about wellness, including skills for monitoring symptoms, decreasing the severity and frequency of symptoms, and improving the quality of life. VOCAL has trained more than 130 recovery facilitators who utilize the WRAP curriculum (described earlier) as a wellness practice. REACH facilitators also work to foster collaboration between service providers and consumers with the goal of increasing their spirit of partnership.

VOCAL Consumer Owned and Operated Programs   The VOCAL Consumer Owned and Operated Programs (CO-OP) is a collection of peer-run, grassroots programs offered throughout the state. It is represented at present by approximately thirty-five programs. VOCAL CO-OP staff and volunteers offer connections and support so peer-run programs can achieve their goals. Toward this end, VOCAL CO-OP offers free publications, consumer scholarships, consultations, workshops, training institutes, program development mini-grants, a website, and information to help create recovery programs.

VOCAL Network   The VOCAL Network promotes connections among individuals and groups across the state with the purposes of increasing individual well-being and allowing support and information to be exchanged. This activity is addressed by connecting inquiring consumers with their peers through linkages with vocational centers, drop-in centers, and support groups. To facilitate these connections, VOCAL maintains a website and Facebook site, and publishes a quarterly newsletter, *Network News*. Organization representatives are selected to serve as communication linkages between VOCAL and specific peer groups, organizations, or localities.

Firewalkers   VOCAL has produced a two-hundred-page volume, *Firewalkers: Madness, Beauty, and Mystery: Radically Rethinking Mental Illness* (VOCAL, 2009) for consumers and professionals that chronicles the experience of severe mental illness through the biographies of seven individuals, whose stories illustrate that recovery is possible for all such persons. The book is sold throughout the state at VOCAL and other related functions.

VOCAL has not undergone formal outcome evaluations, but monitors its impact by tracking the numbers of consumers it serves and the number of initiatives that result from its consultations, activities, and trainings.

National Alliance for the Mentally Ill

The above two program examples are grassroots in origin, having emerged from the initiatives of consumer advocates. It must be mentioned, too, that established organizations like the National Alliance for the Mentally Ill (NAMI) also facilitate consumer leadership opportunities in service delivery. Three such opportunities are described next.

The Peer-to-Peer Support Group   In the Peer-to-Peer Support Group, trained consumers provide education and support services to other consumers in such areas as understanding the nature of mental disorders, stigma, discrimination, relapse prevention, relationship development, decision making, empowerment, and coping strategies.

The Family-to-Family Program   The Family-to-Family Program is a structured education and support program consisting of twelve classes in which trained families with more experience present information to their peers.

In Our Own Voice   In Our Own Voice is a ninety-minute stigma-reduction program whereby one or two consumers with a particular mental illness give community presentations as a means of educating both professionals and lay persons, and sensitizing them to the nature of mental illness.

A Social Work Model of Recovery Practice

In this section, a guiding model of recovery practice is presented for social workers; it is similar to existing models of clinical case management (Walsh, 2009). As we have seen, the values of the social work profession are consistent with those of the recovery philosophy, so there is no need to reinvent the wheel.

Traditional case management practice, from which some recovery models are partly derived, is an approach to social services delivery in which the social worker focuses on the development of growth-enhancing environmental supports for consumers, utilizing resources that are spread across agency systems (Surber, 1994). Clinical case management is additionally characterized by a social worker's addressing relationships among the biological, psychological, social, and environmental factors that influence the course of a person's mental illness and life (Wong, 2006). That is, clinical case management attends to the psychosocial (internal) needs of a consumer and facilitates environmental supports.

Although recovery-oriented social work practice (referred to as recovery practice from this point forward) incorporates most elements of case management practice, it places a greater emphasis on partnerships with consumers and attention to their holistic needs and desires. Recovery practice is particularly appropriate with consumers who have serious mental illnesses such as schizophrenia, major depression, bipolar disorder, and substance use disorders, because these conditions present consumers with continuous or intermittent challenges as they work toward a desired quality of life. Consumers may need assistance with developing self-esteem, self-confidence, self-efficacy, social relationships, housing, income supports, medical care, job training, recreation, life skills development, counseling, and medication monitoring.

While the individual nature of recovery practice does not easily lend itself to large-scale evaluation studies, various types of case management have been found to be effective with regard to helping consumers with mental illnesses function satisfactorily in community settings of their choice (Essock et al., 2006). Many case management programs attempt to uphold values of the recovery philosophy of mental illness, but others are lacking in this regard. A recent study of consumer, family, and staff from sixty-seven ACT teams in Ontario found that recovery activities were only partly upheld, and that some teams were perceived by consumers as being overly directive in their practices (Kidd et al., 2011).

Characteristics of Recovery Practice

Recovery practitioners use a bio-psycho-social stress-vulnerability model to understand the interplay of forces that influence the quality of a consumer's life. In every situation, the social worker combines the sensitivity and interpersonal skill of the psychotherapist with the creativity and action orientation of the environmental architect (Walsh, 2009). As a model of practice, recovery does not prescribe particular intervention strategies, because these will always emerge from each consumer's needs and preferences. Nevertheless, recovery practice always gives priority to the quality of the relationship between the consumer and the social worker as a prerequisite for assisting with the consumer's personal growth. Due to the inherent problems with role confusion and authority in traditional case management practice, where practitioners may be spread across several agency systems, it is further assumed that the consumer is best served when the social worker functions as the primary therapeutic resource.

Recovery practice includes eleven activities within three general areas of focus, as adapted from Kanter (1996, 2006):

1. The initial phase includes the tasks of consumer engagement (including outreach), assessment, and intervention planning.
2. The consumer focus includes intermittent individual psychotherapy, living and coping skills development, and psychoeducation.
3. An environmental focus involves linking consumers with community resources, consulting with families and other caregivers, expanding social networks, collaborating with physicians and hospitals, and promoting consumer advocacy.

The full range of the social worker's range of activities within this model will be described in the next chapter, with a more detailed focus on the nature of its interventions.

Tasks and Activities of the Recovery Practitioner   Recovery practice requires that the social worker serve as the consumer's collaborator, and help the consumer achieve whatever life goals he or she prioritizes. Harris and Bergman (1988) have summarized the major tasks of social workers engaged in clinical case management practice (which extends to recovery) as follows:

- Make a positive connection, and develop a facilitative relationship, with the consumer. This process may unfold in a variety of ways depending on a particular consumer's characteristics and needs, and may range from high levels of interaction to the maintenance of interpersonal formality and distance.
- Model adaptive and growth-enhancing behaviors to facilitate a consumer's movement from a position of service system dependence to one of greater self-direction. When this process is successful, the consumer comes to understand that he or she has unique needs, goals, and skills, and that focused actions can influence the course of events toward achieving specific goals.
- Alter the consumer's physical environment through processes of resource creation, facilitation, and adjustment. These activities speak to the social worker's environmental activities.

Chapter 5 is devoted to an elaboration of the first of these tasks, but some basic points about the importance of the relationship are highlighted next.

The Importance of the Social Worker–Consumer Relationship   The social worker–consumer relationship provides a critical context for positive outcomes in all recovery practice situations. This alliance consists of a positive emotional bond between the parties, mutual comfort, and a shared understanding of goals and related activities. It develops over time in unpredictable ways from the expectations, beliefs, and knowledge that each person brings to the relationship. Several researchers (e.g., Miller et al., 2005) have found that the quality of the working alliance is more predictive of positive outcomes in direct practice than any other variable. The recovery relationship provides an environment of safety for the consumer, and within that context the consumer can

- Develop an appreciation for greater lifestyle structure,
- Appreciate the significance of internal and external limits for improving impulse control,
- Learn that formal and informal help is available for most problems in living,
- Improve reality testing,
- Experience new learning, and
- Enhance self-esteem and self-direction through success experiences.

In short, the recovery relationship provides a context in which the full range of medical, rehabilitative, educational, social, and spiritual interventions can be effectively implemented.

Therapeutic Skills for Recovery Practitioners   In addition to relationship-building skills, social workers need to possess psychotherapy skills in recovery practice, because they might be working with consumers over a long period, through successes and failures, on goal-directed activities. Social workers need not subscribe to any particular theories of intervention, but in the course of their work they will need to make careful judgments in the following areas (Harris & Bergman, 1988; Kanter, 1995, 1996):

- Titrating the appropriate level of worker activity at various stages of the consumer's recovery process
- Continually assessing a consumer's fluctuating competence and changing needs over time
- Differentiating the biological, psychological, and social aspects of mental illness
- Recognizing a consumer's conscious and unconscious motives for behavior, and how these may at times be in conflict
- Developing a longitudinal view of the consumer's strengths, limitations, and symptoms
- Determining when to withdraw support to maximize a consumer's capacity for self-directed behavior

- Helping significant others, such as family and friends, understand the perspectives of the consumer, when indicated

Some program developers are reluctant to support community-based recovery practice due to concerns that social workers may focus too much on psychotherapy practice in lieu of the full range of case management interventions (Neugeboren, 1996). Achieving such a balance is challenging for social workers, and underscores the need for ongoing professional development and supervision. The practice of psychotherapy also demands that social workers engage in ongoing reflection and self-awareness activities toward the goal of understanding their own biases about a consumer's potential for recovery, as described below.

Professional Stigma   While all social workers are expected to adhere to the values of individual dignity, self-determination, and social justice, they may nonetheless hold, perhaps unconsciously, some biased negative assumptions about consumers' social functioning potentials (Lysaker, Buck, & Lintner 2009). This professional stigma refers to the ways in which a social worker's own inclinations to unduly perceive consumers as having certain upper limits for recovery may affect the nature of his or her interventions. With such an attitude, a social worker may, for example, discourage consumers from applying for a certain type of volunteer or work position, believing that the goal may be unrealistic in the context of the mental illness. Another way that a practitioner's own stigma may be displayed is assuming that some consumers can only succeed with exceptional support efforts on the social worker's part, leading to overly benevolent gestures that foster dependency. Clearly, it would be inappropriate for a recovery practitioner to support all of a consumer's inclinations; professional judgment is one of the important services that the social worker can provide. Still, social workers need to continuously reflect on the extent to which their reservations about consumers might be based on stereotypical assumptions rather than on comprehensive assessments of each consumer.

Likewise, social workers must be aware that consumers may experience self-stigma—that is, self-doubt that arises from internalizing social attitudes, and perhaps those of significant others, about their limitations or growth potential. The recovery philosophy was developed by consumers who were able to transcend these limiting social attitudes, but ours is still a society that tends to see mental illness in a negative light. Many consumers who are determined to achieve a high quality of life may nonetheless deal with serious insecurities related to their sensitivity to the attitudes of others.

Now that the basic principles of recovery-oriented practice have been described, an illustration of the process is provided to demonstrate how the practice can be implemented.

An Example of Recovery Practice

The Expectant Couple

Nancy Duncan was a twenty-five-year-old married, pregnant, Caucasian female, unemployed and living with her husband Roger, who was out of town on business several days a week. Roger contacted the mental health center at the suggestion of a friend and told the agency that his wife had a "problem with irrational thinking." He said the same problem had resulted in a brief psychiatric hospitalization in another city when she was twenty-one years old. At that time, Nancy had expressed incapacitating fears of molestation by a vaguely defined "gang," which was in fact nonexistent. When her delusions, as they were diagnosed, were prominent, Nancy would not leave her home or even go upstairs in her townhouse when alone, for fear that she might be assaulted. She experienced these fears only occasionally; overall her perceptions appeared to be normal and Nancy was described as "a great, fun person" who could attend to most of her own needs. The irrational thoughts never fully disappeared, and became more pronounced when her anxiety increased. Roger added that his wife had been the victim of an armed robbery when she was sixteen, and he wondered if this might be the source of her fears. Still, Roger appeared to have little understanding of his wife's problem and hoped someone would "help it to go away."

At the time of Roger's call, Nancy was five months pregnant; she and her husband were both excited about the pregnancy. Her irrational fears had become more pronounced during the pregnancy, though, and it seemed that Nancy's physical changes, apprehensions about motherhood, and perhaps other life changes might be contributing to her growing anxiety.

Initial Intervention Phase

Nancy was a willing consumer, and she and her husband came to the mental health center for an assessment. The practitioner, whose work was recovery focused, was able to engage the Duncans in a positive relationship rather quickly due to their strong motivation for help. He asked them to clarify what they wanted to address, but they differed on this point: Nancy was convinced of the reality of her harassment. When asked about her goals, Nancy stated that she wanted the people harassing her to leave her alone, wanted to feel more self-confident when at home and in the neighborhood, and wanted to adequately prepare for parenthood along with her husband. The social worker was careful to clarify several times whether these were in fact Nancy's goals, to make sure he was not influencing her choices in some way. He asked how long the Duncans imagined utilizing his services, and they replied that they hoped everything would be "in order" for them once the baby was born. The social worker reviewed the various ways in which he might work with the couple, reviewing a range of reflective, cognitive, behavioral, family systems, solution-focused, and support service referral approaches. The couple agreed on a solution-focused, short-term approach, given their desire to be self-sufficient by the time the baby was born. They did, however, want to consider medication as an option for Nancy, and they were interested in any service referrals for prenatal care that the social worker might recommend.

The social worker identified both Nancy and Roger as the consumer system in this case. Roger agreed with the second and third of Nancy's goals, but he did not acknowledge the reality of the first goal. The social worker suggested a restatement of the first goal: "Nancy wanted to understand more clearly if and why she would be a target of harassment." She and Roger accepted that restatement. With the social worker's lead, given the couple's poor understanding of the area's service system, they agreed on interventions that included a medication evaluation, couples counseling to better structure their support for one another, individual counseling for Nancy at home so she could learn lifestyle strategies for feeling more secure, and a service referral for prenatal care. In particular, Nancy welcomed the medication evaluation as potential relief from her anxiety. The relationship among the three was off to a good start, although it would be tested over the next several months.

Environmental Focus

The social worker provided the Duncans with information about some affordable community prenatal services, and the couple successfully followed through with those recommendations on their own. Other environmental services will be described under the "consumer/environment" section.

Consumer Focus

The social worker arranged for Nancy to receive a medication evaluation at the agency several days later, and he consulted with the agency psychiatrist prior to Nancy's visit. He shared that Nancy had been successfully treated for her delusional ideas in the past with mild doses of antipsychotic medication, but because she was pregnant, this may not be advisable at this time. The physician was not willing to prescribe any drugs to a pregnant woman, making clear his concerns about the vulnerability of her child. When the physician shared these concerns with the Duncans, who both attended the session, along with the social worker, Nancy became upset and stated that she desperately needed relief from her "nervousness." The social worker advocated for Nancy's having regular appointments with the physician, despite the fact that she would not be prescribed medication, and the doctor agreed to see her every two weeks. He added that if the situation became dire, such as the client feeling suicidal, which seemed like a possibility, he might relent and prescribe medication.

Both Roger and Nancy eventually accepted the physician's point of view, but as Nancy's fears increased during the next month, she began to plead with the doctor for medication, and both she and her husband begged the social worker to "do something" to relieve her stress. This was an example of two professionals opposing the consumer's stated preference because of their concerns for the physical safety of a child. Relationships between the Duncans and social worker became strained as a result, although they still agreed to meet with him and the physician as scheduled.

Nancy appreciated the social worker's twice-weekly, thirty-minute visits to her townhouse. While they were of opposite genders and approximately the same age, the social worker did not experience any boundary concerns during his home visits because Nancy always behaved in a pleasant but formal manner, and focused all conversation on her own family. The social worker in turn was task-focused in helping Nancy develop a daily structure that felt safe to her. He understood that Nancy was most anxious when alone, and that when others were present she could relax and focus her attention away from her fears. During their conversations, the social worker articulated Nancy's many strengths as a wife and mother-to-be, and supported her hopes that her fears would eventually be resolved. He also gently challenged the rationality of her thinking. Nancy became less sure of the reality of her harassment, and wondered if perhaps she was overly sensitive to her husband's being at work or traveling. Nancy's delusional thinking persisted through the following four months but, with the social worker's support, became less pronounced; he taught Nancy some relaxation strategies that benefited her.

A new challenge to the quality of their working relationship developed when Nancy began calling the social worker at his office once or twice daily for reassurance. The worker had invited Nancy to do this once per week on a particular day and time, but his failure to initially uphold a strict limit on this practice proved to be a mistake. Nancy, who often felt she was in crisis, began calling more and more frequently, and soon was keeping the agency receptionists on the line several times per day, asking them for help when the social worker was not available. (Indeed, the receptionists had a meeting with the social worker and his supervisor to air their concerns.) The social worker finally set firm limits on Nancy's calls, but they were difficult to stop. Nancy became frustrated, and rightfully expressed anger at the social worker's lack of consistency. In retrospect, the social worker concluded that his initial invitation to Nancy to call had been disempowering of her, making her feel more reliant on the agency than she perhaps needed to be.

The Duncans met with the social worker weekly at his office for couples counseling. The stress that had increased since Nancy's pregnancy had put strains on their relationship. As much as they cared about each other, Roger was not sure how to respond to his wife's continuous needs for reassurance. During their meetings, the social worker provided education to the couple about the nature of irrational thinking and its relationship to anxiety; he was careful not to use the term "delusions." By this time, Nancy was not opposed to such discussions. The social worker introduced the couple to the idea of behavioral exchange as a theme of their work together. That is, both spouses might benefit from a shared task of learning how they could concretely be more supportive of each other's positions. Prior to their agency involvement, Nancy had experienced major blows to her sense of self-efficacy in the marriage, and Roger had developed a pattern of quick rescue behaviors, about which he was now becoming frustrated. The social worker helped the couple to more clearly delineate their shared roles within the household. This was particularly helpful to Roger, who was beginning to feel that his wife's potential to manage the household was limited, when in fact she had many strengths and much good judgment to bring to the couple's domestic and financial situations. It was during the couple's sessions that the social worker was able to recapture some of the goodwill that had characterized their earlier sessions.

The social worker was aware during this time that his psychosocial interventions alone would not help Nancy achieve all her goals. However, he believed they were useful for helping the Duncans through the pregnancy, after which time medication could be utilized. Furthermore, his cognitive interventions seemed to be helpful in encouraging Nancy to question the validity of some of her perceptions. Again, the social worker never suggested outright that her perceptions were wrong.

Consumer–Environment Focus

After learning that Nancy had a support system in the area (mother-in-law, sister-in-law, cousin, and friend), the social worker suggested that the Duncans try to structure Nancy's days by inviting some of them to visit her on a regular basis; she was not comfortable driving. The couple invited these four people to separate meetings with the social worker and, from the perspective of supporting Nancy as a new mother-to-be, they set up a schedule of visits so that Nancy was rarely alone for a full day. This routine helped Nancy to contain her fears. The social worker reminded Nancy that she needed to maintain primary responsibility for her designated household and pre-natal care responsibilities.

Five months after Roger's first call, Nancy gave birth to a healthy girl. Soon afterward, the social worker referred her to the physician for another medication evaluation, and she agreed to take a low-dose antipsychotic drug. The medications were help-ful, and Nancy's affect stabilized significantly. Still, although she enjoyed motherhood, her fears of being in public alone per-sisted. Nancy called her husband at work several times a day even though he usually came home for lunch. When he was out of town, she called and often visited with her relatives and friends.

The social worker had concerns about the ongoing extreme caregiving behaviors of Nancy's support system and devoted the last few of their sessions to a discussion of the issue. The worker pointed out that Nancy's strengths might be best nur-tured if she developed a greater ability to tolerate being alone. She might enjoy the mobility, and the freedom from relying on the schedules of others. Furthermore, he explained, other fam-ily members and friends, as helpful as they were, might grow to resent spending so much time with her. The couple agreed, Nancy a bit reluctantly, and designed a plan for weaning Nancy from the frequency of her visitors.

Despite Nancy's ongoing moderate anxiety, the baby was doing well, and she and Roger were doing well as parents. The couple soon decided to end their involvement with the social worker, believing they were getting along well and could handle the family situation on their own. Nancy transferred responsibility for her medication to her own family physician. The end of the intervention, five months after its beginning, seemed appropriate. Nancy and Roger had achieved their goals. The social worker reminded them, however, that Nancy should give ongoing attention to her anxiety issues, and that they could return to the agency if they desired professional assistance in the future.

Intervention Summary

At the beginning of this intervention Nancy was not consciously involved in a recovery process, because she, unlike her husband, had not accepted that she was dealing with a long-term mental illness. The social worker hoped that as a result of their work together Nancy might come to accept that she had a condition requiring ongoing attention, and continue on a recovery journey. The social worker provided recovery-oriented interventions: he was collaborative with the couple, attended to Nancy's biological, psychological, and social concerns (reflecting the recovery value of holism), followed her lead in goal setting, and set a process in motion by which the Duncans could carry on with their own intervention after he was no longer present in their lives (empowerment).

The social worker was careful to collaborate with the couple and elicit choices from them (self-determination) about the various services from which they might choose. He constructed an individualized service plan (individual action) with input from the couple and physician, and he consciously worked from a strengths basis in determining what resources and supports were available to them.

While the couple largely achieved their goals, the five-month intervention included several points of conflict among the parties involved. The social worker and physician acted in ways they believed were ethical while exercising their power in making some decisions, such as withholding medication and limiting phone calls (limiting consumer self-direction). The social worker sought informed consent (demonstrating respect) from the consumers at every step along the way, and was largely accepting of their perception of the nature of Nancy's problems. He provided input into the process but gave them the responsibility of managing their support systems and continuing their adaptive behaviors when the intervention ended. Nancy seemed aware that she would need to continuously monitor her mental status and social functioning, and thus she and her husband understood that her recovery process would be ongoing.

In his work with the Duncans, the social worker did not utilize a structured, standardized measure of goals and objectives, but rather used numerous consumer-focused measures that are available for use in recovery practice that may facilitate the process, as described below.

Goal Setting in Recovery Practice

A consumer's desired recovery outcomes may be different from those typically identified by helping professionals. Recovery from mental illness represents an interactive process that involves transactions between the person and his or her support systems, treatment system, and community (Loveland, Randall, & Corrigan, 2005). Mental health practitioners and researchers have tended to focus more narrowly on symptom outcomes. Anderson, Caputi, and Oades (2006) identified desired outcome differences between professionals and consumers by reviewing a sample of measures with 281 consumers. The professionally developed criteria tended to focus on behaviors, symptoms, self-care compliance, and measures of impairment, social functioning, and withdrawal. Consumer-generated recovery measures, however, focused on their feelings about themselves and their levels of fucntioning, and their attitudes about the resources to which they have access.

Goal-Setting Instruments

The instruments described next represent efforts to prioritize consumer perspectives in the goal-setting process.

Goal Instrument for Quality   The developers of the CRM discussed earlier in this chapter introduced a formal review instrument known as the Goal Instrument for Quality (Clarke et al., 2009). This template is not for writing goals and objectives, but rather for evaluating their quality. The instrument is noteworthy in its emphasis that each set of goals and objectives should begin with a statement of the consumer's vision—that is, the hopes, dreams, and values from which all other elements of the plan derive. Other desired elements of appropriate goals and objectives are said to include

- Evidence of social worker–consumer collaboration,
- Clear behavioral definitions,
- Consumer ratings of perceived goal importance,
- Ratings of consumer confidence or self-efficacy with regard to each goal
- Specific time frames for goal accomplishment,
- Periodic indications of levels of goal attainment,
- Presence of an action plan,
- Identification of possible obstacles, with a prevention plan,
- Attention to social support, and
- Evidence of regular goal monitoring.

In a study of 122 practitioner files in eastern Australia, the same authors found that a vision statement was most often missing from goal formulations; evidence of active goal monitoring was also missing. They found, however, that practitioners became more attentive to these elements with training.

The Recovery Assessment Scale   The Recovery Assessment Scale (Corrigan, Salzer, Ralph, Sangster, & Keck, 2004) is a forty-one-item, five-point Likert scale that summarizes consumer outcomes in the areas of personal confidence and hope, a willingness to ask for help when needed, personal goal and success orientation, appropriate reliance on others, and not being dominated by symptoms.

The Mental Health Recovery Measure   The Mental Health Recovery Measure (Young & Ensing, 1999) is also a forty-one-item, five-point Likert scale, and evaluates a consumer's recovery in the areas of overcoming stuckness, discovering and fostering self-empowerment, learning and self-redefinition, returning to basic functioning, striving to attain overall well-being, and striving to reach new potentials.

Recovery Process Inventory   The twenty-two-item Recovery Process Inventory (Jerrell, Cousins, & Roberts, 2006) is an interview survey that evaluates consumer outcomes with regard to the six factors of anguish, connection to others, confidence or purpose, care from others, living situation, and self-care or hopefulness.

Stages of Recovery   The Stages of Recovery instrument is a fifty-item survey that addresses ten significant areas of recovery (Anderson et al., 2006). Those authors assert that consumers identify recovery as a developmental process including the five stages of moratorium, awareness, preparation, rebuilding, and growth. With this instrument, respondents are asked to designate their current stage of recovery from among the five choices, and then to rate each item with regard to their associated feelings of hope, responsibility, identity, and meaning on a six-point scale.

Canadian Occupational Performance Measure   The Canadian Occupational Performance Measure (COPM) defines the term "occupation" as the everyday tasks in which a consumer engages that are both culturally and personally meaningful (Kirsch & Cockburn, 2009). The measure incorporates a semistructured interview that is carried out in four steps: (1) delineation with the consumer of any occupations that are perceived as challenging in the areas of activities of daily living, productivity, and leisure; (2) consumer ratings of the importance of each activity; (3) consumer ranking of his or her five most important occupations and level of satisfaction with them; and (4) periodic reassessment of identified occupations and the consumer's score on both performance and satisfaction.

Whereas all of these recovery measures have been evaluated for utility and effectiveness with promising results, more research is required before their overall validity and reliability can be established (Loveland et al., 2005).

To conclude this discussion of recovery practice, it is important to consider the routine worker or client boundary challenges that arise as the parties attempt to work together collaboratively.

Boundary Issues in Recovery Practice

In recovery practice, the social worker and consumer may interact in a variety of community settings. When these interactions take place, the social worker often develops relationships with the consumers' friends, family members, landlords, employers, and other helping professionals. The scope and intensity of intervention challenges the social worker's ability to develop appropriate relationships with consumers. Considering relationship issues from the perspective of boundaries provides an important source of guidance for the social worker.

Boundaries are the assumed, and often unspoken, rules that people internalize about the physical and emotional limits of their relationships with others. They protect one's privacy and reflect his or her individuality. Through boundaries, people organize their social worlds and communicate their positions within them. People differentially construct their boundaries to facilitate their desires to be close to or separate from others. They open and close boundaries to control the flow of their interactions. Each person's boundaries are unique, overtly and covertly communicated to suit their assumptions and intentions about particular relationships.

Boundary-making begins as early as six months of age, when infants first develop a sense of separateness from parent figures (Gabbard & Lester, 1995). Boundaries continue to develop through life, and the ways in which they are constructed become more stable over time. It is considered healthy to be flexible in boundary setting, because this promotes a person's ability to adapt to changing relationships and environments.

A person's social and personal characteristics determine some of his or her boundaries (Wallace, 1997). People may be included with or excluded from other groups based on, for example, their gender, race, ethnicity, class, position in a hierarchy, and cultural traditions. Boundary patterns are also reflected in personality types. The person with rigid boundaries tends to be intolerant of ambiguity, to have a high internal locus of control, to value predictable behavior, and to be controlling, confrontational, and guarded. The person who maintains flexible boundaries desires autonomy but is adaptable, arbitrative, and open. The person with fluid boundaries, which is not a desirable trait, is tolerant of ambiguity but has a high external locus of control, tending to be impulsive and needing to be liked by others.

So how does the recovery practitioner negotiate this aspect of relationships with consumers? Curtis and Hodge (1994) state, "If community workers are not facing relationship boundary issues in their daily work, they are probably not doing their jobs most effectively" (p. 341). The nature of recovery practice, with the social worker providing services in the consumer's territories, ensures that boundary dilemmas will frequently emerge. For that reason, social workers need to be careful in both establishing interpersonal boundaries and deciding when those boundaries can be crossed. When these issues are openly addressed and boundaries are consistently negotiated, consumers will be more willing to participate in the helping process. Mutually understood boundaries provide an appropriate sense of control, power, protection, self-determination, and, above all, trust for both consumers and social workers. Any practitioner actions perceived by consumers to be transgressions of interpersonal boundaries, intentional or not, may have negative consequences for the relationship. Consumers may feel exploited, disrespected, or controlled (Gutheil & Gabbard, 1998). In extreme circumstances, such as inappropriate physical contact, boundary transgressions can have legal consequences for the worker.

Boundary establishment is important to the professional survival of recovery-oriented social workers—indeed, to all practitioners (Farber, Novack, & O'Brient, 1997). Clear boundaries are healthy for social workers because they promote role clarity regarding the range and limits of intervention activities, a basis from which to make decisions about how and when to cross physical or psychological boundaries, and physical safety (when territorial boundaries are maintained). Boundaries are healthy for consumers, as well, because they promote a relationship in which the consumer feels affirmed and respected, a predictable environment in which the consumer is more likely to feel comfortable sharing personal information at his or her own pace, a sense of individuality and self-determination that derives from having control over boundaries, and a basis from which to determine whether and when the social worker can cross certain boundaries.

The Nature of Social Worker–Consumer Boundaries

In recovery practice, boundaries include rules about the following aspects of relationships:

- Contact time. How much time is appropriate for the social worker to spend in the company of the consumer? Will contact time vary depending on whether it is spent face to face, on the phone, online, or otherwise? Will it vary depending on the time of day, day of the week, or time of the year, or on the purpose of the contact?
- Types of information to be shared. What is the appropriate range of topics for the social worker to discuss with the consumer? Is information limited to job topics or social topics? What about politics, religion, and sex? How much depth can the social worker be expected to provide about these topics?
- Physical closeness when together. What are the social worker's expectations about personal space when in the consumer's company? How close together should they sit? Are certain forms of eye contact not appropriate? Can the social worker touch the client, and vice versa? What range of nonverbal communications is appropriate?
- Territoriality. To which of the consumer's environmental spaces does the social worker have access? From which is he or she restricted? Can meetings be held at the consumer's home? Can they be held at the social worker's home? Should interactions be limited to social settings? Recreational settings? The agency office?
- Emotional space. To what extent should the social worker be willing to share feelings about sensitive topics with the consumer? Is it appropriate for the social worker to share feelings of personal sadness, trauma, and anger at others?

Crossing Boundaries

The discussion thus far has focused on boundaries as limits, but the concept also has implications for bridging and access (Petronio, Ellemers, Giles, & Gallois, 1998). All people experience natural tensions to remain apart from and to join with others, and this underscores the importance of flexibility in boundaries. Boundary crossing refers to appropriate efforts to adjust boundaries toward greater intimacy, while boundary violations are inappropriate entries into a person's privacy and space (Hermansson, 1997). As examples, boundary crossing might involve a social worker's efforts to gradually talk with a consumer about appropriate but intimate details of his personal life, while a boundary violation might involve an abrupt effort to connect with a withdrawn client by shaking her hand, patting her on the back, or offering a hug. Another example of a boundary violation is prematurely assuming that a consumer approves of home visits.

People decide whom to let in as well as whom to keep out. In most relationships that persist, boundaries change. People test the boundaries of others to determine how they should behave toward them, and if and when they can move closer. If a person attempts to cross a boundary about which the other person is not comfortable, the latter may choose to withdraw, and perhaps erect new, tighter boundaries in response. In the long-term nature of much recovery practice, it is likely that worker–client boundaries will evolve. Crossing them may be appropriate, but violating them is not.

Boundaries and Power

Boundary awareness is particularly important in recovery practice because, despite their collaborative efforts, power differentials do exist between the two parties. Social workers control certain material and emotional resources needed by the consumer, and the consumer must be (or thinks he or she must be) compliant with the worker's agency-sanctioned procedures to qualify for those resources. This lack of equal power in the relationship may compromise the consumer's ability to defend him- or herself with regard to privacy issues. Some social workers fail to see how their power may stir the consumer's resentment in times of negotiation or disagreement. A consumer will only loosen a boundary when he or she perceives some benefit to doing so, however, and he or she needs to trust the worker and feel confident that the relationship will be enriched as a result of doing so.

Warning Signs of Possible Boundary Transgressions

Possible boundary transgressions that may emerge in the course of recovery practice are described next. None of these is necessarily a transgression; whether it is so depends on particular circumstances, which will be considered in the next section.

- Intrusion into the consumer's territory. The high utilization of home visits provides one example of how community care has shifted the balance of power to the consumer in some ways. The home represents a private territory in which persons can exercise control and expect visitors to abide by their rules (Bruhn, Levine, & Levine, 1993). Intrusive activity includes visiting the consumer who does not want to be visited or making unannounced home visits, both of which are commonplace (for example, in child protective services work).

- Most dual relationships, or those in which the social worker interacts with the consumer or the consumer's significant others, in more than one role (Herlihy & Corey, 1997). For example, the consumer or significant other might be the social worker's mechanic, grocer, neighbor, fellow church member, and so on. These situations create potential conflicts of interest as well as opportunities for confidentiality violations. They are most common in rural settings, but can occur anywhere.

- Self-disclosure by the social worker. This practice may be legitimate at times as a means to a therapeutic end, but it may also involve a sharing of personal information for the worker's benefit. A social worker who shares that he had an argument with his son that morning may be using the consumer as a resource for venting. This may put the consumer in the inappropriate position of being a caregiver.

- Socializing with consumers. The boundary between intervention and socialization (talking about issues that are unrelated to the purposes of the interaction) is often difficult to distinguish in recovery practice. A social worker may be invited to a consumer's graduation ceremony, a family's holiday cookout, or a party planned by a group of consumers. These may be appropriate shared activities, depending on what the social worker communicates in doing so. Sometimes, however, the social worker may spend too much time socializing with a consumer, even during a contact that is task-specific. While informal communication is useful for establishing a relationship and building a consumer's social skills, it may indicate that the social worker is attending to his or her own needs, rather than to those of the client.

- Referring to consumers as friends. Social workers rarely interact with consumers in the same manner as they do with their friends. With friends, people tend to be self-disclosive about their weaknesses and fears, and are willing to sacrifice personal time to offer assistance, loan money, and give advice about personal matters. Communicating to consumers that they are friends is misleading. It may cause eventual hurt feelings or discourage consumers from developing their own friends.

- Investigating irrelevant details of consumers' personal lives (Doreen, 1998). The need to know some personal information about consumers does not mean that the social worker has a right to know everything. The social worker's curiosity may be voyeuristic at times (for example, with regard to a consumer's sexual practices).
- Loaning, trading, or selling items to a consumer. This includes such practices as lending money, trading compact discs, or buying and selling items such as artwork and furniture.
- Accepting or giving gifts. This may or may not be appropriate, depending on the consumer's and worker's motivations, the nature of the relationship, and the material value of the gift. It may be an important action to help consumers practice reciprocity in relationships (expressing gratitude for assistance, for example). Often, agencies have policies that the social worker must follow to establish limits in this area.

Social workers should also monitor their countertransference reactions to consumers, which represent responses to consumers based on conscious and unconscious personal feelings. These reactions will be discussed in chapter 5.

Other Factors in Considering Possible Boundary Violations

The preceding list consists of possible, not actual, boundary violations. A variety of other factors must be considered when assessing the nature of the social worker's boundary conduct (Curtis & Hodge, 1994). These include

- The consumer's ability to use appropriate judgment in interpersonal situations;
- The consumer's history in relationships (his or her ability to manage conflicts, closeness, or differences of opinion);
- The history and dynamics of the particular relationship (what patterns of interaction have been established, and whether a

boundary-crossing activity by the worker is likely to be growth-enhancing or a setback for the consumer);
- Cultural norms reflected in the behaviors of both the worker and consumer;
- Legal liabilities that the social worker might face by engaging in certain actions; and
- The social worker's consideration of principles from the NASW Code of Ethics (2008).

A Word About Boundaries and Professional Groups

The social worker's ability to successfully coordinate interventions for consumers also necessitates clear boundaries with other professionals. As with social workers and consumers, members of professional groups maintain boundaries between themselves and other such groups, marked by different bodies of knowledge, language, values, histories, and intervention preferences. For physicians, psychologists, social workers, and nurses, boundaries demark their realms of expertise.

Issues of power among the professions have consequences for the quality of consumer care (Petronio et al., 1998). Professionals tend to assert that the problems relating to their specialty should be kept within their domain. Psychiatrists are licensed to prescribe medication, and they may not welcome members of other professional groups giving input into that process. Psychologists have expertise in psychological testing, and they may not accept that social workers have adequate diagnostic expertise. These interprofessional boundaries present challenges to recovery practitioners, who may need to coordinate services among a variety of professionals while sometimes being excluded from the decision-making activities of those persons. While frustrating at times, these boundaries need to be negotiated as best as possible, because separation from other professional staff may result in social workers restricting their case consultation activities, and thus failing to benefit from the input of other professionals in ensuring optimal services for consumers.

Managing Boundary Dilemmas

Listed below are guidelines that social workers and supervisors can follow to help them reflect on boundary dilemmas in recovery practice.

Guidelines for Social Workers

- Set clear boundaries with consumers at the beginning of those relationships about what the social worker's roles and activities will and will not include. Consumers should participate in establishing these boundaries.
- Clarify boundaries with the consumer over time, because they will change. For example, the social worker and consumer may decide that home visits that have not yet been made are now indicated, or that they will address a broader or narrower scope of the consumer's issues than was done initially.
- Consider the preservation of the consumer's privacy as a major guiding value. The social worker should always reflect on how much he or she needs to know about a consumer, and what the purposes are of acquiring certain information.
- Be aware of one's own emotional and physical needs as much as possible, and be wary of obtaining too much personal gratification at the expense of a consumer. If a social worker's personal life goes through periods of unhappiness, he or she may unwittingly look to consumers too much as a source of validation.
- Always promote the psychological separateness of the consumer (Simon & Williams, 1999). All activities should be focused on the goal of making the consumer more self-sufficient rather than dependent on the social worker.
- Be educated about the consumer's cultural and community standards of behavior, so as to understand what boundaries are reasonable in those contexts (Herlihy & Corey, 1997).
- Use peer consultation and formal supervision routinely.

Guidelines for Supervisors

Most important, supervisors should provide a safe forum for worker disclosure. Because many boundary dilemmas are related to the social worker's personal feelings about consumers, they are not always easy to discuss with a supervisor (or anyone else). The supervisor can be sensitive to the worker's personal situation and help him or her differentiate normal emotional reactions from feelings that promote boundary violations. Supervisors should be proactive in identifying and evaluating typical boundary dilemmas that occur in practice, which will bolster social workers' confidence that their supervisors are open to discussing them. Social workers should not be concerned that an admission of a boundary dilemma will put his or her job or reputation at risk. It is a sign of maturity when a social worker admits to uncertainty about how to manage relationships with some consumers.

Discussions of boundary dilemmas should proceed as a process of guided exploration rather than cross-examination (Gutheil & Gabbard, 1998). In guided exploration, the supervisor helps the social worker to reflect on and resolve his or her boundary concerns in an atmosphere of support and affirmation. A supervisor's attitude of confrontation or cross-examination puts the social worker on the defensive and discourages the processing of dilemmas. Additionally, supervisors should promote clarity in recovery workers' job descriptions. Recovery practice is stressful, in part because boundaries for both parties can seem blurred. With role clarity, social workers will have an easier time deciding what is or is not appropriate in their activities with consumers.

Summary

Recovery has emerged during the past twenty years or more as a significant philosophy for helping consumers holistically manage and perhaps transcend their mental illnesses. Specific program models for recovery, generated by professionals and consumers, are now in use in many mental-health-care systems. Federal and state governments have taken initiatives in promoting this change in service philosophy, although it has been left to providers to develop these ideas. The programs developed by professionals and consumers appear to complement each other, and consumers have demonstrated that they have unique service contributions to make in bettering the lives of their peers.

The model of recovery-oriented social work practice presented in this chapter provides a basis from which social workers can collaborate with and support consumers as they work toward their recovery goals. This model, which is highly consistent with the profession's person-in-environment perspective, is based on a clinical case management approach to practice. The social worker utilizes psychosocial skills for counseling persons with mental illness but also draws from an extensive knowledge of community systems to help consumers develop a range of formal and informal supports toward their goals of optimizing social functioning and facilitating an orientation to recovery as a long-term project.

Recovery practice goes beyond clinical case management in its deliberate adherence to the recovery philosophy of mental illness, in which priority is placed on partnership with, collaboration with, and empowerment of the consumer, who is always encouraged to be self-directive with his or her recovery plans. The social worker must be prepared to act as a consumer advocate in securing resources from agencies and other professional groups, some of which may place less value on the recovery philosophy.

Social workers may be challenged to develop appropriate relationships and interpersonal boundaries with consumers. The boundaries of their interactions must be openly negotiated and reviewed over time so the social worker can maintain a focus on goals that are consumer centered.

Major Chapter Learning Points

- A practice model is a concrete guiding strategy for human services professionals to follow in providing recovery-oriented services, or for consumers to follow in their own recovery processes.
- The ability of direct practice social workers to engage in recovery practice must be facilitated and supported by policies of the service system in which they are used.
- A variety of recovery-focused intervention models have been developed by professionals and consumers, examples of which include the Collaborative Recovery Model (CRM) and the Illness Management and Recovery Model (IMR) (professionals); and the Wellness Recovery Action Plan (WRAP) and Virginia Organization of Consumers Advocating Leadership (VOCAL) (consumers).
- Recovery practice in social work is characterized by attention to recovery values; a collaborative relationship between the social worker and consumer systems; holistic attention to biological, psychological, and social aspects of recovery; and a utilization of consumer-generated outcomes.

- A variety of formal measures of recovery outcomes for consumers are available for use by social workers, although their validity and reliability are still being tested.
- Boundaries are the assumed, often unspoken, rules that people internalize about the physical and emotional limits of their relationships with others. The scope and intensity of recovery intervention challenges the social worker's ability to develop appropriate boundaries with consumers.

Questions for Reflection or Discussion

1. Consider the benefits and risks (if any) of employing peer specialists on community treatment teams.
2. Are there elements of models of recovery practice that can be incorporated into your practice in the absence of formal adoption of any models?
3. What are the various strengths and limitations of the five recovery outcome measures described briefly in this chapter? Does one appeal to you? Why?
4. Consider boundary dilemmas you have faced in your personal or professional life. Did you handle them well? Is there anything you might have done differently to prevent interpersonal conflict from developing?

Chapter 5

Relationship-Based Intervention with Recovering Consumers

The following comes from Elliot, a twenty-seven-year-old single African American male who has schizoaffective disorder:

> I'm the type of person who, when I have a problem, it all comes undone. So if I have a small problem it's like waiting for the sun to go down, like it's gonna just explode, and come undone, and there are parts I just have to clean up in the morning. A lot of people my age, they're waiting for the sun. . . . It's like Japan, land of the rising sun, it's like they've been out for so long they're just waiting for a new day to dawn. I'm not like that, people are not like that, some of them don't know it's a fantasy. Sometimes I don't know, or forget whether I should talk about my friends who have screwed up, if it's important to go over those things, or if I should focus on happier things. It can be important. . . . I have a lot of issues.

Much of the practice literature is focused on how social workers can engage with persons who are psychotic after they have stabilized and can communicate in conventional ways. It is true that social workers and consumers may have difficulty at times understanding each other, which can frustrate their mutual efforts to form a relationship. Still, consumers can be engaged in working relationships even when their symptoms are prominent. A social worker's relationship-development skills in recovery practice are thus important because they represent one of the nonspecific elements of intervention. The purpose of this chapter is to examine the range of nonspecific elements of intervention, the nature of communication of persons who are psychotic, and principles for social workers to engage those persons in positive relationships. With this information it is hoped that social workers will be able to more effectively connect with their consumers toward the goal of initiating recovery interventions.

Nonspecific Aspects of Professional Intervention

As discussed in chapter 2, professional technique is not the only variable that accounts for consumer outcomes, regardless of the person's presenting diagnosis. In fact, five factors that influence treatment outcomes have been identified in one literature review (Spaulding & Nolting, 2006) as including

1. Consumer characteristics,
2. Events that occur outside the formal intervention setting,
3. Relationship factors,
4. The consumer's expectancy of receiving help, and
5. The practitioner's intervention techniques.

The value of therapeutic relationships is widely acknowledged but is still the subject of debate within the helping professions (Furman, 2009). Some practitioners believe that a good relationship is sufficient for consumer change, while others assert that therapeutic technique is more important. Hewitt and Coffey (2005) conducted a meta-analysis of studies on the significance of the social worker's relationship with consumers who have schizophrenia and concluded that consumers who experience an empathic, positive relationship with a provider have better outcomes. Additionally, Miller and colleagues (2005) concluded from their literature review that the two elements of the therapeutic alliance and the practitioner's ongoing attention to the consumer's attitude about the intervention account for positive outcomes more than any other factor. They estimated that consumer characteristics (the nature of problems, motivation, and participation) account for 40 percent of intervention outcome, the quality of the therapeutic alliance accounts for an additional 30 percent, the practitioner's guiding theory or model accounts for 15 percent, and the remaining 15 percent is a placebo effect.

Frank and Frank (1993) engaged in a worldwide study of the determinants of positive outcomes for all persons who seek the assistance of helping professionals. They concluded that the following elements were predictive of positive outcomes; several of these speak to the quality of the relationship:

- The consumer enters into an emotionally charged relationship with the provider, and perceives that person to be competent and caring.

- The provider has confidence in whatever theories and techniques he or she utilizes.
- Interventions are based on a rationale that is understandable to the consumer.
- Interventions require the active participation of both the provider and the consumer.
- The provider gives the consumer opportunities for learning and success experiences.

Most recently, Norcross and Wampold (2011) summarized the findings of an American Psychological Association Task Force on Evidence-Based Therapy Relationships, which consisted of a series of research meta-analyses conducted by panels of experts. Among their conclusions were these:

- The relationship makes substantial contributions to an outcome independent of the specific type of treatment.
- The relationship accounts for why clients improve (or fail to improve) at least as much as does the particular treatment method.
- Practice guidelines should explicitly address therapist behaviors and qualities that promote a facilitative relationship.
- Efforts to promulgate best practices or EBPs without including the relationship are seriously incomplete.
- Adapting or tailoring the therapy relationship to specific consumer characteristics enhances the effectiveness of treatment.

The task force concluded that there was most research support for the variables of therapeutic alliance, empathy, and regularly collecting client feedback. Activities around goal consensus, collaboration, and positive regard were deemed "probably efficacious," while genuineness, repairing relationship ruptures, and managing countertransference were "promising" factors that lacked strong research support.

The remainder of this chapter will elaborate on the significance of relationship-based factors in recovery intervention.

Thought and Communications in Psychosis

There is no single definition of psychosis, but it can be understood as a mental state in which external reality has a diminished meaning for an individual or is perceived in a highly unconventional way (Campbell,

2004). The core of psychosis is characterized by thought blocking, thought deprivation, poverty of thought, and loose associations. The periphery of psychosis, or the ways in which the core is manifested, may include hallucinations (auditory, visual, tactile, olfactory, somatic), affective impairments (flat, blunted, social withdrawal, noncommunicative, passivity, ambivalence), delusions (persecution, thought broadcasting, thought insertion, thought withdrawal, being controlled, being the focus of external events, somatic distortions, grandiosity), and loose speech (tangential responses, loss of a goal, or seemingly purposeless and illogical associations) (APA, 2000). Even in psychosis, however, the person can make many rational observations and choices, and retain his or her strengths and talents (Taylor, 1997).

The Experience of Psychosis

Psychotic ideation may be evident in many disorders, both medical and psychiatric, including thought disorders (schizophrenia, schizoaffective disorder, delusional disorders), and mood disorders (major depression, bipolar disorder), among others (APA, 2000).

Thought Disorders

The thinking and perceptual distortions in psychosis result from neurological changes, the origins of which are not clear. These include disruptions in the person's short-term memory and information processing capacity, which are related to impairments in stimulus filtering (Cadenhead & Braff, 2000; Keefe, 2000). An overload of normally inhibited stimuli leads to the person's misinterpretation of words and events. This in turn leads to an impairment in executive functions, which normally allow a person to plan, organize, follow sequences, and think abstractly (Palmer & Heaton, 2000).

The perceptions of persons with thought disorders feature a loosening of the commonsense visual and auditory fields (Uhlhaas & Mishara, 2007). Whereas a person's visual field normally perceives objects in meaningful relationship to one another, the loosening of perceptions separates out and highlights fragments from the larger context. The individual perceives partial elements of a scene without grasping its overall meaning. This phenomenon produces delusions, as the person struggles to find coherence in his or her fragmented perceptions. These perceptual processes are often manifested by odd speech patterns (Harvey, 2000). Auditory hallucinations are in turn the result of mental processes that are experienced as detached from their internal source.

An example may illustrate this point. A socially isolated consumer with schizophrenia lost himself in religious fantasies, based on fragmented perceptions of his family's actual belief system. Without the ability to make sense of his distorted perceptions, and in the context of his loneliness and anxiety, he constructed a story that he perceived as being sensible that he had been sent to earth by God, doomed to suffer in isolation for the betterment of mankind. He had the gift of being able to interpret evil messages hidden in popular music, and took as his mission the warning of others that they were being brainwashed by Satan. In this way, he composed a view of his world that he perceived as being coherent, that included an important place for himself.

Below is another example of a confused communication from Elliot about conflict with his family:

> I'm heading toward the wilderness. I understand what it means to go south. I'm just naturally heading out of town. Sometimes I have to go to town, and it's not a big deal because I never plan to stay. I'm perpetually working to get out of town. My family is always trying to get to town, and I'm trying to get out of town. Going into town is always exciting for me. Most people go into town, they see subways, they see New Japanese, and they're stuck there for a week. They have to get work done. I'm in and then out. I don't spend money there. It's a different attitude.

Mood Disorders

In major depression and bipolar disorder, a person's thinking style and behavior are at the mercy of uncontrollable moods (Goss, 2006). When depressed, one's thinking is slower than normal and relatively lacking in focus. During the experiences of hypomania and mania, the person's elation is accompanied by a loss of control over his or her thoughts. In hypomania, a moderate amount of elation may actually sharpen one's cognitive abilities, but speech and thought can degenerate into psychosis during mania. Manic persons cannot complete thoughts because the affective rush propels them cognitively in different directions, as evidenced in the following example of Sarah, a consumer who was expressing resentment of her successful younger brother, a computer engineer:

> They're actually making computer chips out of sand from the beach. That's two huge work issues; organic versus sustainable. Like, you can't rip down the rain forest, but you can extract plants from it. Well, why are you allowed to go in if you aren't allowed to touch anything? But organic, a lot of men argue, "What is inorganic?" A problem to a psychologist is some idiot did heroin and fused both halves of his brain together; how do you get them apart? You can't open it up. It's like a person, you can't open him up.

Sarah, who was a bright, articulate woman, started out with a certain idea, although its nature is not at all clear, but her out-of-control mood state drew that thought into this direction, and then that direction. Not only was she unable to complete a coherent thought, but she also lost track of the original idea.

The Potential for Connection

While the presence of psychosis presents challenges for the social worker in relationship development, it also provides opportunities. The consumer with psychosis often feels marginalized and discounted by others, so any evidence of the social worker's acceptance will be perceived and eventually welcomed. Furthermore, the person with psychosis does not completely lose his or her understanding of social conventions (Arieti, 1974). Much of the social worker's early intervention may involve helping the consumer to place perceptual fragments into a wider, more cohesive context (Roberts, 1997).

The recovery interventions described next, which are an elaboration of points featured in chapter 4, emphasize the use of the relationship in helping consumers develop improved attachments toward others and an enhanced awareness of the social contexts that can facilitate their goal attainment.

Intervention Guidelines

There is a long history in the psychotherapy literature on the importance of relationship development with consumers who experience psychosis. Semrad (1955) argued that empathic connection with psychotic persons is critical for their improvement, and that the emotional connection between consumer and practitioner can help mitigate the consumer's sense of isolation. Sullivan (1947) wrote that a lengthy interpersonal relationship is required to shed light on the psychotic consumer's difficulties in living, because the consumer cannot always communicate his or her way of life well. Havens (1996) characterized the social worker–consumer relationship as a sanctuary that attempts to balance the consumer's conflicting desires for solitude and society. Weiden and Havens (1994) outlined obstacles that may interfere with therapeutic alliance development with persons who have schizophrenia, including their suspiciousness of others, sense of stigma and demoralization, and terror from the experience of symptoms. The interpersonal strategies that can help to ameliorate these obstacles include empathizing with the fear, providing alternative points of view, making affirming statements, and normalizing the experience of stigma.

What follows are guidelines for relationship-based interventions that can help consumers progress through the early stages of recovery. The first is ongoing, while the others unfold in a sequential manner.

Sustainment

Sustainment is an intervention that summarizes the ideas introduced above. The social worker–consumer relationship is the sustaining link between the recovering consumer and social worlds, and provides the consumer with an environment of safety. When it is positive, the consumer becomes aware that the social worker appreciates the threads of meaning in his or her fragmentary statements (Cox, 1997). The consumer's cautiously trusting response to being understood facilitates his or her movement in the direction of personal integration, adaptive functioning, and general recovery.

The social worker sustains and enhances the recovering consumer's sense of self through verbal and nonverbal interventions, by

- Listening actively and sympathetically,
- Conveying a continuing attitude of goodwill,
- Expressing confidence and esteem,
- Reassuring the consumer about his or her recovery potential, and
- Offering environmental support (Goldstein, 1995).

The social worker promotes a confiding relationship and instills in the consumer a sense of competence and caring. The social worker's presence becomes an antidote to the consumer's alienation, inspires the expectation of help, and creates a setting where constructive confrontation can eventually take place. Within this relationship, the consumer improves his or her perceptual accuracy and experiences enhanced self-esteem.

In the following statement, Elliot expresses faith in his relationship with the social worker:

> Does counseling help? Not in the sense of my daily life. But it helps with my routine. If I have a problem I know I'll have an answer when I'm here, so I can make a note, a mental note, so if I have some work to get done, if I have something to say, and it's intense, I can say it in a scientific manner, and use my psychology. I trust that this is a real outlet. I've learned from experience that a degree is useful to have, and it reinforces that there is an answer. Where science is cold, a scientific person will not be offended by a scientific answer.

The social worker often cannot initially comprehend what a psychotic consumer is saying, and any quick attempts at interpretation may amount to free association on the practitioner's part. The sustaining social worker thus should not rush to interpret the recovering consumer's comments (suggesting "this" really means "that"), but rather should accept them with curiosity ("this" means "this," but perhaps also "that"). The possibility of eventual success in building the relationship may be diminished by quick interventions: recovery is a lengthy process and the consumer may choose to not become engaged in a partnership with the social worker.

The remaining intervention guidelines are adapted from Dilks, Tasker, and Wren (2008).

Expanding the Consumer's Perspective

Effective communication with psychotic consumers requires that the social worker gradually perceive the meaning of the consumer's seemingly bizarre statements. Toward that end, the social worker gradually encourages the recovering consumer to elaborate on his or her thoughts regarding areas of concern. The social worker anchors the consumer's statements and beliefs in social contexts that run counter to the consumer's sense of isolation. That is, the social worker first attends to the context of disclosure, offering feedback as an outside observer, while seeking to understand the consumer's inner world and content of disclosure. The social worker does not argue for or against the objective reality of a consumer's beliefs, but explores the feelings behind them, and slowly begins to adjust his or her sustaining responses to include other possibilities (perhaps "this" means "that"). This process respects the consumer's need to set the pace of recovery.

As an example of this process, the social worker's response to Elliot's confusing statement is included below. It is important to emphasize that the social worker was only able to formulate his idea of the meaning of Elliot's statement (anxiety about being scrutinized by others) after spending several weeks getting to know him.

> Elliot: Eye color . . . when I was in college eye color got really important, I can talk about it. Apparently in adolescence your eye color can change, but it doesn't permanently change. My eyes look green sometimes when they were brown my whole life. And some people are really overly intense with eye color, in college, and eye contact is intense, so when you start making eye contact. . . . I'm comfortable with you, but some teachers are really big on it. It's not like high school where you can really get out of order, and I really have a bad reaction to staring. And I can be intimidating because I'm an athlete. My personality is, I'm the kind of person who can bring up an eye contact discussion. But you can't do that everyday in class.

> The social worker: I get the impression, Elliot, that it's hard for you to be around other people, especially strangers. They might look you in the eye, and intrude on your space, and make you nervous. It seems like when people try to get physically close to you, or talk to you, you get uncomfortable.

Processing Distress

The social worker regulates the emotional pace of the intervention by structuring conversations to minimize the possibility of the consumer becoming overwhelmed by negative feelings. With the social worker's acceptance and support, the consumer can stand back from distressing experiences or concerns so he is no longer overwhelmed by them. The consumer's modulated distress can then become the object of sustained discussions.

> Elliot: My mom, brother, and dad are all into sweets, desserts and stuff like that, and I'm not. Things that are nice look sweet. A lot of things that look nice are not sweet, like bananas, that have a

lot of vitamins, and jam has a lot of sugar. So they tend to walk all over me at times. They'll gang up on me to get what they want. They'll let me go hungry, it's a dissention [*sic*] problem. Here I can just spill my guts. My parents don't like it, nobody believes me. Here I can just say it, and I won't hear "just let it go." Whatever I say in here, it's just a topic. I can decipher feelings, and I don't want to feel people getting confused.

The social worker: So you can't relate to your family very well. They often seem to be on a different page than you are, so to speak. And it seems to upset you that you feel so isolated, and maybe sometimes you wonder if something is wrong with you because of this. But Elliot, you have a right to your feelings; everyone does.

Facilitating New Understandings of Situations

The social worker repeatedly observing and empathizing with the consumer's experiences and concerns can move the consumer toward considering alternative conclusions regarding his or her perceptions. The social worker filling in perceptual gaps provides the consumer with new possibilities for assessing and reacting to his or her concerns. If the consumer trusts the social worker, he or she will consider this input and reconsider the nature of his or her experiences, opening up possibilities for functioning differently.

Elliot: I keep getting into trouble with the police. There are a lot of shady characters in my neighborhood, and I'm pretty sure they're selling drugs. I see these people all the time, just hanging out. So I call the police. But last week the police wound up coming to my house again, and complaining to my dad that I was causing trouble. But I'm in the neighborhood most of the time, and other people aren't, so I see what goes on better than most people. And there's a police officer living just two doors down. I think he moved in to monitor the crime situation. Lately I've been filing my reports with him, but that guy called my dad, too.

The social worker: Elliot, you've told me you haven't actually seen these people dealing drugs. Maybe they're just people who are hanging out. If they look suspicious, it doesn't necessarily mean that they're doing anything wrong, you know?

Introducing New Possibilities for Action in the Social World

This summary strategy involves the social worker's encouraging and supporting the consumer's elaboration of activities, meanings, and life goals. If the consumer perceives the social worker to be a concerned listener and trusted assessor of the consumer's position in the social world, he or she will feel more grounded about making recovery plans (Walsh, 2000). The consumer can develop a new self-understanding based on a more thorough integration of past and present concerns (Rhodes & Jakes, 2009).

Elliot believed that he was destined to be a great Olympic athlete, specializing in cycling events. Since his initial psychotic break in late adolescence, and after he had become socially isolated as a result of that episode, he found solace in taking his bicycle into the countryside for long rides. He was very much an amateur in this sense, but the activity supported the development of a belief that he was preparing for the Olympic games. This goal had been a theme throughout their work together and the social worker never argued against it. Rather, he encouraged Elliot to share his training regimens and other preparations, and only gradually suggested that he explore alternative plans for his current and future life. The social worker emphasized that it was a good idea for anyone to have back-up career plans in case his primary goal did not work out. What follows are Elliot's thoughts about changing his career goal. It is apparent that he is considering a more social life for himself:

> Elliot: I can always be a cyclist, no matter what. I can practice around here if I get my own apartment, and enter the local and regional events like I already do. It might be less expensive if I don't turn professional, and I could spend time doing other things. I've worked in restaurants, you know, and I like cooking, so maybe I'll become a professional cook. I've cooked at home a lot. It makes me feel less guilty about still living at home. Cooking can be a career, and it can also be something you do for friends. I'm no good with girls, they seem to be put off by me, I don't know why, but maybe if I cooked for them, I'd have a chance. I could ask them out, and when they say, "What will we do?" I'll say I can cook for them. And then we can have something to talk about, which is my cooking the meal.

Whether Elliot had the talent and focus to get through culinary school, which became his new career goal, remained to be seen. But it was a more realistic goal for his personal growth potential than professional athletics. Soon after making this decision, he found a job in a sandwich shop.

Thus far we have been focusing on the challenges of relationship development without considering in depth the social worker's and consumer's personal feelings about, and reactions to, one another. These feelings, commonly known as transference and countertransference, can be subtle in their influence of the quality of worker–consumer interactions. In the following section, we review the potentially positive and negative effects of the social worker's countertransference feelings when working with consumers who have psychotic symptoms.

Transference and Countertransference in Recovery Practice

The concepts of transference and countertransference have been prominent within psychodynamic theory since its beginnings, and have extended into other practice theories to some degree (Gabbard, 1995). Transference was initially defined as a consumer's unconscious projection of feelings and wishes onto the practitioner, who comes to represent a person from the consumer's past such as a parent, sibling, or other relative (Jacobs, 1999). The social worker may not actually possess those characteristics, but the consumer acts as if he or she does. The concept has gradually expanded to refer more broadly to all reactions that a consumer has to the social worker, based on patterns of interaction with similar people in the consumer's past or on actual characteristics of the practitioner. In positive transference, the consumer is attracted to the practitioner, which can facilitate the clinical engagement process. Negative transference is characterized by such feelings as anger, distrust, or fear, all of which impede the consumer's participation in the interaction.

Countertransference was initially defined as a practitioner's unconscious reactions to the consumer's transference projections (Jacobs, 1999; Kocan, 1988), but the concept has also broadened to refer to the effects of the practitioner's conscious and unconscious feelings on his or her understanding of the consumer. The social worker's countertransference reactions are based on his or her personal history, values, biases, attitudes, anxieties, self-concept, protective instincts, and cultural background (Mandell, 2008). These feelings are often best understood in hindsight, with reflection, since they are partly unconscious. Countertransference reactions should be taken into account in every practice encounter with regard to how they influence the social worker's perception of a consumer. The social worker's awareness of his or her emotional reactions facilitates the consumer's recovery process, because it helps the practitioner better understand the reasons behind his or her words and actions.

Transference and countertransference reactions can be best understood as relational, mutually influenced by the ongoing exchanges between the consumer and social worker (Knapp, 2003). Another term, cotransference, might better capture the intersubjective aspect of the social worker's participation with the consumer to mutually influence each other's reactions (Goldstein, Miehls, & Ringel, 2009).

When examining his or her countertransference, the social worker should reflect on the following six questions (Mandell, 2008):

1. What person or persons does the consumer remind me of?
2. Which of my own painful experiences is being stirred by our work?
3. What judgments am I making about the consumer, based on my personal values?
4. What was I hoping to accomplish by making a (certain) comment or asking a (certain) question?
5. Are my behaviors congruent with the consumer's goals and the principles that inform my practice approach?
6. If I could act (experience some situation again), would I do the same thing?

Some characteristics of social workers that may produce problematic countertransferences include the need to be needed, liked, and in control; the need to feel like an expert; being uncomfortable with certain kinds of emotional expression; and overidentifying with consumers whose problems are similar to one's own (Kocan, 1988; Schoenwolf, 1993). Specific countertransference reactions include dreading or eagerly anticipating seeing a consumer, thinking excessively about a consumer when away from work, having trouble understanding a consumer's problems, being bored or unduly impressed with a consumer, feeling angry with a consumer for nonspecific reasons, feeling hurt by a consumer's criticisms, doing things for the consumer that he or she is capable of doing, and feeling uncomfortable when discussing certain topics. These reactions are only problematic when they cause the practitioner's decision making to be based on his or her feelings rather than on the recovering consumer's goals. In a sense, consumers offer social workers an opportunity for emotional development through understanding aspects of themselves that they find most challenging.

Countertransference and Intervention Outcomes

Ideas about countertransference (like transference) have primarily arisen out of case studies, but recent meta-analyses of the literaure have assessed its impact on intervention outcomes in more systematic ways (Hayes, Gelso, & Hummel, 2011). The first meta-analysis (of seventeen studies) indicated that countertransference reactions are related inversely and modestly to psychotherapy outcomes, and another (seven studies) revealed that managing countertransference successfully is related to better therapy outcomes. The authors conclude their review with the following statements:

- The effective practitioner can manage countertransference reactions in ways that benefit the work.
- The practitioner's struggle to gain self understanding and work on his or her own psychological health are fundamental to managing his or her internal reactions.
- Self-integration underscores the importance of the practitioner resolving his or her major conflicts that may affect practice, which points to the potential value of clinical supervision.

Countertransference and Schizophrenia

Transference with persons who have schizophrenia is often unstable. The social worker steps into an ambivalent consumer's world and must be prepared for his or her mixed emotions (Post, 1982). The consumer has needs for interpersonal connection, but at the same time fears putting trust in others (Savage, 1987). The social worker may in turn have negative feelings about the consumer because the work is sometimes unrewarding, and the practitioner may project his or her own ambivalence about the work onto the consumer (Walsh, 2000). The social worker's emotional distancing from the consumer may serve as a defense against these negative reactions.

Several research studies provide examples of consumer-induced countertransference with persons who have schizophrenia. One study found that practitioners experienced such consumers as submissive and friendly during the early stage of intervention (Schwartz, Smith, & Chopko, 2007). Another comparative study found that practitioners experienced consumers with schizophrenia as more interesting and less frustrating, but also more provoking of anxiety and hopelessness, than consumers with depression and borderline personality disorder (Brody & Farber, 1996). Hassan, Cinq-Mars, and Sigman (2000) wrote a revealing article about countertransference issues that emerged among the coleaders of a schizophrenia therapy group when conflict emerged among the members. All three practitioners stifled their own anger during the conflict situation because of their shared wish to help members relate in a secure atmosphere, and because of their perceptions of the members' fragility. They resisted any expressions of anger among the consumers and later recognized that this might have led to inappropriate actions on their part. One coleader's desire to encourage nonconflicted behavior exacerbated her own frustration, and she admitted that as the mother of a large family she usually felt compelled to extinguish arguments.

We now turn to an extended example of a partially failed attempt to provide recovery interventions in which many of the chapter themes are illustrated.

Barry's Ambivalence

Barry was a twenty-five-year-old unemployed African American male with schizophrenia. He was of average height and slightly overweight, and with thinning prematurely grey hair he looked older than his years. Barry lived with his mother, who held a full-time job, in a suburban neighborhood of a Midwestern city. His parents were divorced and his father lived a few hundred miles away. Barry was referred to the mental health agency from a psychiatric hospital where he had spent several days following a suicide attempt. He had been treated at the same hospital for several weeks three months before his assignment, during his first active episode of schizophrenia.

Barry was assigned to an agency social worker named Robert, a married Caucasian male just a few years older than the consumer, whose position was that of a clinical case manager. Robert would be responsible for Barry's individual therapy and his linkages to an agency physician and appropriate community service providers. The social worker's agency did not formally incorporate a recovery model of practice, but Robert's own practice values included working collaboratively on consumer-generated goals related to a satisfactory overall lifestyle. Robert was proud of his reputation as the agency expert on psychotic disorders, and he was very good at engaging consumers in comfortable working relationships. His meetings with Barry would be held at the agency.

While reviewing the referral information, Robert learned that Barry had been extremely withdrawn throughout his adolescence and early adulthood, gradually retreating from family and peers. He attended high school and adequately managed his basic activities of daily living, but otherwise stayed at home. In late adolescence, Barry began to experience auditory hallucinations, including one soothing and one threatening voice, and tactile hallucinations, including the feelings of being stroked on the leg and of being suffocated while trying to sleep. Barry eventually became so depressed and fearful about these delusions that he was hospitalized. He retained insight into his former self and knew that he was changing in ways that terrified him.

An unusual problem confronting Robert from the beginning was Barry's apparent discomfort with their relationship. The consumer presented as an angry person who perceived others as unhelpful and nonsupportive. Robert sensed that Barry was not invested in their work together, and this bothered him. Robert was confused because he had a reputation of being sensitive to psychotic consumers' feelings of isolation, and they usually responded well to his empathic presence. But Barry was different. Robert's initial (and unconscious) reaction to this situation was to feel angry with Barry, and he withdrew a degree of his typical empathy and emotional support. Robert tended to (more consciously) blame Barry for his lack of follow-through with therapy tasks (even calling this behavior passive aggressive) rather than try to understand the consumer's ambivalence.

Robert remained unaware of his negative countertransference until his supervisor pointed it out during a weekly group supervision meeting. The supervisor suggested that Barry had a negative interpersonal style with most people in his life, so while this may have been predictable with the social worker, it was difficult for Robert not to take Barry's presentation personally, and as evidence of his ineffectiveness. The supervisor speculated that the social worker's needs to be liked and perceived as an expert were contributing to the tensions between them. Robert's supervisor also knew that the social worker was generally uncomfortable with any consumer's expressions of anger. Barry could be demanding, hostile, and briefly drop out of treatment at times as a means of expressing negative feelings about the intervention plan or his own perceived inadequacies. Furthermore, Barry seemed to resent that the practitioner could not do more for him. The supervisor suggested that Robert was taking offense that the consumer "didn't appreciate" his efforts—but it wasn't the consumer's job to do that! The supervisor assigned Robert to reflect on Mandell's (2008) six questions (described above, this chapter) related to assessing countertransference. After doing so, Robert came to the following conclusions:

- Barry reminded Robert of his peers from adolescence and young adulthood who were harsh and intimidating toward him; Barry and Robert were about the same age.
- As a result of these reminders, Robert's own fears of inadequacy, this time as a practitioner, were surfacing.
- Robert was acting in passive-aggressive ways by making negative judgments about Barry as being unappreciative and uncooperative.

- Robert's withdrawal represented his effort to protect himself from feelings of inadequacy but was inappropriate to the consumer's needs.
- Robert's expectation that Barry assume so much responsibility for his own level of treatment participation was opposed to the social worker's usual stance of providing much emotional support for recovering consumers.

Robert was upset at these insights, but nevertheless decided that he needed to act differently, to see Barry as a unique consumer with certain coping behaviors, and to provide him with support that was more active.

The intervention continued, and Barry made slow progress. Barry had identified three major goals in his recovery vision, which he seemed motivated to achieve: getting a good-paying job, finding his own apartment, and meeting enough people that he could find a few male friends. These goals were ambitious, but realistic if Barry pursued them patiently. The social worker was able to maintain a constructive, if somewhat formal, relationship with his consumer. Robert linked Barry with a psychiatrist who developed an effective medication regimen after months of trial and error. The medications controlled, but did not eliminate, his anxiety and hallucinations, and they did little to alter his anhedonia and ambivalence. Next, the social worker enrolled Barry in a computer-training program that lasted for one year and ended with his referral to a job placement agency. Barry's other activities, facilitated by the social worker, included participation in a clubhouse program where he could enhance his interpersonal skills and participate in a volunteer position to test his work readiness. Robert met with Barry every two weeks for counseling and as a central point of case management. After two years, Barry eventually achieved a level of competence and self-esteem where he could look for a private sector job. Throughout their work together Robert encouraged Barry to view his recovery as a life-long process, and to attend to his personal interests as much as his occupational goals.

Robert's relationship with Barry again became conflicted when the consumer, while preparing for regular employment, began to miss appointments, was slow to follow through with referrals, and was slow to communicate his thoughts to the social worker. Robert noticed that he was becoming frustrated again by his apparent inability to help Barry talk openly about his thoughts and emotions. The social worker confronted Barry about his passive behavior at times, noticing that he was falling back into his own angry patterns, but Barry tended to sit quietly and share little. He stared at the clock, ruminated about his lonely social life, and wondered openly if Robert could ever truly understand a person with schizophrenia. The social worker decided to present his consumer to the supervision group again.

Robert believed that he had resolved his relationship issues with Barry, but another colleague suggested the possibility of projective identification. The colleague, who had listened to Robert talk about his challenges with Barry over time, suggested that the consumer had difficulty communicating his fears of relapse and failure. The colleague noted that Robert often expressed similar feelings—that he was ambivalent about the consumer's potential, unsure of Barry's ability to maintain motivation, and concerned about his relapse. Furthermore, Robert felt angry with Barry because he did not seem to want to be helped—but perhaps Barry himself felt angry about the social worker's inability to help the consumer? The social worker's assumptions that Barry was an angry, defensive man might have prevented him from considering that Barry was unconsciously behaving in such a way that the social worker might pick up on his fears. Robert was stunned at his colleague's observation, but realized it was valid.

Robert addressed the issue of projective identification with Barry, although he did not use that term, and the consumer agreed that they seemed to be experiencing the same negative feelings. This was late in the therapy process, however, and Robert worried that his revelation might have come to him too late to be of benefit to his work with the consumer. Robert's concerns about Barry's interpersonal limitations proved to be justified when the consumer attempted suicide a second time several months later. At that time, Barry was despairing over problems managing the responsibilities of a new job—the first one, really, that represented independence. Success on this job might have led to his acquisition of an apartment and responsibility for his own budget. Barry was not functioning well on the job and, lacking adequate social supports, feared that there was no hope for him to succeed. Fortunately, the suicide attempt was not successful. Barry quickly recovered physically but decided to move from the area to live with a relative in a rural environment.

Robert was uncomfortable with the outcome of the intervention. On the one hand, Barry had achieved a number of gains and demonstrated that he could handle the rigors of an intensive rehabilitation program. He accepted that he had a mental illness that would require ongoing monitoring, but he also understood that he had generally good judgment about working with his strengths to achieve his personal goals. On the other hand, Robert's negative countertransference, which had characterized much of the intervention, had seriously undermined his potential to help the consumer process his feelings about the intervention. Robert wondered about the extent to which his frustrations contributed to the consumer's ongoing ambivalence.

Summary

Elliot: Who you are as a person is more important that what psychological organization you are born with.

The quality of the social worker–consumer relationship is critical in working with persons who have psychotic disorders. Only by developing a greater appreciation for the lived experience of consumers can social workers maximize their potential to effectively implement the interventions of sustainment, expanding the consumer's perspectives, processing distress, facilitating new understandings, and introducing new possibilities for action in the social world. These interventions can be useful for ameliorating the psychotic consumer's symptoms and facilitating long-term intervention toward holistic recovery. Implementing these relationship-based interventions is not easy, however, as many consumers at least initially have little faith in relationships. Relevant skills for social workers to develop, so that their potential for connection with consumers might be maximized, include assessing for the effects of cognitive deficits related to psychosis, and the principles of consumer engagement discussed in this chapter.

The social worker's examination of the sources of his or her feelings about consumers reveals much about the quality of the relationship and can help the practitioner better understand the reasons behind his or her actions during an intervention. Countertransference reactions to consumers are often characterized by practitioner discomfort due to the special challenges the social worker experiences in engaging with the consumer. The self-aware social worker can monitor his or her countertransference by maintaining awareness of his or her own emotional needs and being wary of wanting to obtain personal gratification at the expense of a consumer.

Before proceeding to detailed examples of how social workers can support the recovery of persons with specific mental illnesses, it is important to consider the role of spirituality, the topic of the next chapter, in that process.

Major Chapter Learning Points

- Relationship-development skills are essential in recovery practice because they represent one of the nonspecific elements of effective intervention.
- Consumers can be engaged in working relationships even when their symptoms are prominent, and those who experience an empathic, positive relationship with a provider have better outcomes.
- The presence of psychosis presents challenges for the social worker in relationship development, but it also provides opportunities. Consumers with psychosis often feel marginalized and discounted, so will welcome evidence of the social worker's acceptance. Furthermore, such consumers do not completely lose their understanding of social conventions.

- The principles of relationship-based intervention include sustainment, expanding the consumer's perspective, processing distress, facilitating new understandings of situations, and introducing new possibilites for action in the social world.
- Transference refers to all reactions that a consumer has to the social worker, based on patterns of interaction with similar people in the consumer's past or on actual characteristics of the practitioner. Countertransference refers to the effects of the practitioner's feelings on his or her understanding of the consumer.
- Countertransference reactions should always be taken into account with regard to how they influence the social worker's perceptions of a consumer. The social worker's awareness of these reactions facilitates the recovery process because it helps the practitioner better understand the reasons behind his or her actions.

Questions for Reflection or Discussion

1. How can a social worker show empathy to a client who is actively psychotic?
2. Given what has been presented in this chapter about the non-specific aspects of intervention, do you think there may be too much attention given in education to strategy or theory?
3. Think of an example where it might be difficult to consistently utilize sustainment with a client over a long period. What would be some likely challenges?
4. With what types of client do you feel most and least comfortable? What does that suggest about your own countertransference tendencies?
5. Consider the case of Barry, and whether the social worker effectively utilized the five elements of relationship-based intervention. How might he have done so more effectively?

Chapter 6

Spiritual Concerns of Recovering Consumers

There's a reason why I went through what I did. It's a spiritual reason. . . . I promised that when I came through this I would share with others that God had helped pull me through. (VOCAL, 2009, p. 108)

If I had never encountered mental health struggles, I might have lived a life that was quite insulated. I might not have broadened my mind. Sometimes we have to go through our own personal hell to come to a place of reckoning. Though I walked through horrible and scary places, I have found a peace in knowing what kindles my spirit. (VOCAL, 2009), p. 135.

Social workers are encouraged to conduct holistic assessments of consumers: the quality of one's social functioning is a product of the interplay of biological, psychological, social, and spiritual forces. In human services practice, however, relatively little attention is given to consumers' spiritual lives. This topic has traditionally been considered outside the scope of professional concern, and to be a personal issue that is best left to the consumer and his or her support community. Attention to consumers' spiritual concerns may be especially important when working with recovering consumers who experience mental disorders, however. For example, spiritual concerns and religiousness have been shown to be highly prevalent in persons with schizophrenia (Mohr et al., 2010). Those persons have experienced major disruptions to their sense of self and as such often dwell openly on concerns related to purpose and meaning in life. Spirituality can help persons with mental illness develop a positive sense of self, decrease the impact of symptoms on their lives, and provide a network of supportive social contacts. It can also, however, be a source of suffering.

There is a rich diversity of spiritual beliefs and expression in the world that needs to be taken into account in the current climate of globalization. At present, the major religions in the United States include Christianity (76.5 percent of the population), Judaism (1.2 percent), Eastern religions (0.9 percent), Islam (0.6 percent), and Buddhism (0.5 percent). Fifteen percent of the population indicates no religion (American Religious Identification Survey, 2009).

The purpose of this chapter is to consider how the recovery-oriented social worker can assess for and, when appropriate, help consumers address their spiritual concerns. Ethical dilemmas that may arise when attending to spirituality will also be addressed.

Defining Spirituality

We define spirituality here as a person's search for and adherence to ultimate meanings, purposes, and commitments in life (Frankl, 1988). People may not deal with these concerns on a daily basis, but when they are faced with loss, identity struggles, estrangement, and the fear of isolation, they often return to them. Furthermore, these ultimate concerns influence how people organize their lives.

As mentioned in chapter 3, spirituality is not the same as religion. In this chapter, both concepts, and the related concept of existentialism, will be subsumed under the term "spirituality." It is understood that these concepts are complex and may be formulated in different ways.

The social work profession has developed an increased awareness of the role of spirituality in recovery for a variety of reasons. These include a recognition of its importance to overall health and coping, the profession's holistic perspectives on human behavior, a greater appreciation of the importance of cultural competence in services provision (sometimes called religio-competence), and increased attention to the voices of consumers, who often describe the significance of spirituality in their recovery processes (Fallott, 2001). Social workers may face difficult ethical dilemmas in this regard as well (Barnett, Jeffrety, & Johnson, 2011). For those clients for whom issues of religion and spirituality are relevant, ethical issues may include when and how to conduct a spiritual assessment, given that others may be more qualified to do so; worker competence with the topic; boundary issues regarding discussions of spirituality; the possible need to coordinate interventions with other professionals; and how to effectively integrate spiritual issues into practice.

The Will to Meaning

In social work, with its strengths perspective, spirituality can be represented by the will to meaning, which represents each person's basic, enduring tendency to obtain what satisfies his or her nature (Frankl,

1988). This perspective assumes that all people have an innate drive to either create or discover meaning and purpose in life. There are no specific meanings to which one should aspire; these are realized through one's passions and interests. There are inherent risks, however, in maintaining a will to meaning. Having a purpose beyond the self includes an awareness of vulnerability and responsibility; and a potential for tragedy, anxiety, and loss in life.

Spiritual meanings can be summarized into four categories, which may overlap. Belief systems may be (1) religious or secular. One can believe in the teachings of the Islam faith because one believes in its divine origins, or in the golden rule (act toward others as you want them to act toward you) because it reflects a human value. (2) Social concerns include commitments to social causes. One can demonstrate such a commitment, for example, in volunteer service of various types, commitments to bettering the quality of life for certain oppressed groups, or actions to address environmental concerns. (3) Creative pursuits include involvement in artistic endeavors, but may also include approaches to one's work, such as the development of innovative agency programs. Also included in this category is the experience of creative pursuits that bring meaning to one's life. Some persons feel most alive, for example, when listening and responding to a piece of music. Finally, (4) hope includes the defiance of suffering. This comes to the forefront of existence at times when one experiences great self-doubt or despair, but recognizes that one values life enough to persist in overcoming the adversity. Hope is, of course, key to the recovery process.

The sharing of some troubling emotions provides signals that consumers are struggling with spiritual concerns (Lazarus & Lazarus, 1994). Most prominently, some types of anxiety result from threats to one's identity, future well-being, or concerns with life and death. This anxiety is fueled by the struggle to maintain a sense of connection to others with the onset and experience of mental illness. The emotion of guilt results from thoughts or actions that people perceive as violations of important social standards of conduct. Guilt results from a perceived moral flaw when one has not behaved in accordance with an important value. A religious person who commits a transgression against a higher power and a social worker who provides poor service to a consumer might both feel guilt. The emotion of shame is similar to that of guilt, but refers more specifically to the failure to live up to a personal, rather than social, ideal. A Caucasian person who believes in equality of opportunity may feel shame when he or she reacts negatively to an African American family moving into the neighborhood. It is important to emphasize that persons experience positive emotions such as happiness and joy when they behave in ways that affirm the spiritual self. A consumer who performs well as a Habitat for Humanity volunteer may experience great joy from making that contribution to the community.

The Importance of Spirituality in the Recovery Process

The experience of psychosis is a deeply personal process. A psychotic episode represents a profound assault on one's personality, identity, self-esteem, and confidence. One author has termed the onset of psychosis as a "spiritual emergency" (Lukoff, 2005, p. 233). The consumer experiences an internal fragmentation that may prompt challenges to his or her quest for life meaning. Spiritual preoccupations can have positive or adverse effects on the consumer (Fallott, 2001). The person may experience grandiosity, frightening delusions and hallucinations, or episodes of major depression due to self-deprecating spiritual beliefs.

Distinctions between psychotic and mystical experiences are not clear-cut (Dein, 2007). In both there is a lessening of the boundary between the self and the outside world, and in the sense of agency (being the initiator of one's actions and experiences). Both are influenced by cultural factors: psychotic experiences that are feared in some cultures are revered in others. In fact, in cultures where the experience of the spiritual or psychotic realm is valued, consumers with mental illness have a better prognosis for recovery (Clarke, 2000). With a functional continuum between normality and psychosis, what professionals consider as the point where a person crosses the threshold is not so much the content of his or her beliefs as it is the consequences (Peters, 2001).

More than seventy years ago, Anton Boisen (1936) outlined characteristics of spirituality, based on his study of hospitalized persons, that have relevance to persons struggling with schizophrenia. He noted that persons experiencing either religious struggles or emotional breakdowns were similar in questioning their identities and their place in the world. He conceptualized their sense of isolation as a state of mind characterized by estrangement from those with whom they formerly sought identification. In a positive way, spirituality provided the (then-called) patients with a sense of identification with a fellowship transcending the self, and helped them to face difficult life situations in light of ultimate values. Others have noted that the outcome of the struggle to recover from schizophrenia depends on the presence or absence of a nucleus of purpose around which a new sense of self can be formed (Imbrie, 1985).

Several qualitative studies provide illustrations of these points. In one study of the experiences of eight consumers, respondents noted that during the onset of their psychosis they experienced great suffering, and sensed that dark, sinister forces were at work, aimed at destroying them (Murphy, 2000). Many of these consumers questioned whether there was any meaning in life. Such questions prompted the consumers to experience depression, but religious faith or spiritual conviction often provided answers to their sense of isolation. Faith and religious practice fostered attitudes that promoted their well-being. Holford (1982), in a naturalistic study of forty-two consumers divided into religious and control groups, investigated the prognostic significance of religious belief. Personal prayer, found to be important to more than half the Holford respondents, was generally used in constructive ways, much as it had been in the person's life prior to the illness. In a similar vein, a national sample of 235 consumers in Canada indicated that prayer, loosely defined, was a major holistic healing practice for enhancing mental health (Russinova et al., 2009). Sullivan (1993) conducted a research project with forty respondents who had a serious mental illness but were, by their own report, functioning successfully. Of these, 48 percent stated that spiritual beliefs were central to their success.

Another quantitative literature review revealed that 80 percent of consumers with psychotic disorders found attention to spiritual and religious issues to be helpful in their recovery process, and only 5 percent reported that this was not a source of support (Lindgren & Coursey, 1995). Spirituality played a positive role in their coping with stress and decision making, enhanced their tangible and emotional support experiences, including their relationships with a higher power, and strengthened their sense of being a whole person. Clearly, social workers should never devalue consumers' spiritual ideation, whether or not it is conventional, because this would be the equivalent of denying part of their existence.

By way of summary, the positive spiritual themes in the recovery stories of consumers in another qualitative study included the following (Fallott, 2001):

- A whole-person spiritual language that helped consumers transcend more-limiting psychiatric labels
- Faith-based perseverance in the recovery journey
- Assurance of hope
- The power of loving relationships, both human and divine
- The experience of serenity
- The promotion of genuineness and authenticity as existential goals
- Participation in spiritually informed activities that express their core beliefs

One caveat in this discussion of spirituality is that, at least among persons with schizophrenia, religious beliefs and attitudes tend to be labile. A three-year follow-up of 115 consumers found that whereas religion was consistent among 63 percent of respondents, it changed in a positive way for 20 percent and in a negative way for 17 percent (Mohr et al., 2010). If a social worker addresses spirituality, he or she should not assume that this area of a consumer's life will be perceived in a consistent manner over time.

Mental health practitioners have often tended to feel uncomfortable or unqualified to address issues of spirituality with consumers, due in part to concerns about imposing their values on them (Sheridan, Bullis, Adcock, Berlin, & Miller, 1992). In a major study in Canada and Switzerland of 221 consumers with psychotic disorders and their 57 providers, researchers found that although religion was an important aspect of their lives, many of the practitioners were unaware of their consumers' religious involvements, even if they reported feeling comfortable with the issue (Borras et al., 2010). Within the same sample, 100 consumers in Geneva and their 34 providers found that 16 percent had positive psychotic symptoms related to aspects of their religious beliefs (Huguelet, Mohr, Borras, Gillierson, & Brandt, 2006). Only 36 percent, however, raised the issue of their religion with their providers. Some of these providers reported that, in their view, religious practice was incompatible with professional intervention. Still, providers were seldom consciously aware of this conflict, and 50 percent of them had inaccurate perceptions of their clients' religious involvements. In a related earlier study of 328 Virginia social workers, Sheridan and Bullis (1991) found that practitioners struggled with the issue of incorporating spirituality into their practice; the same spiritual interventions were considered to be appropriate and inappropriate in equal numbers by the respondents.

Examples of Consumers' Spiritual Orientations

The following two vignettes illustrate different ways in which consumers may integrate their spiritual inclinations into the process of coming to terms with mental illness.

A Rainbow

Harold is a forty-year-old single African American male with schizophrenia, featuring prominent paranoia. He lives with his sister and her young son, but they have a distant, conflicted relationship. Harold is always hyper vigilant and feels harassed; he is tormented by degrading auditory hallucinations. He is routinely barred from public places for angrily confronting innocent others he accuses of verbally abusing him. He also confronts his social worker regularly for allegedly thinking ill of him, or expressing dislike in nonverbal ways. Many people consider Harold to be potentially violent, although he has never physically assaulted anyone.

Harold had a Baptist upbringing but now has no formal church affiliation. His religious beliefs, which no other professional had asked him about, are surprising in the context of his behavior. When invited by his social worker to elaborate on the topic of his religion, he said, "I think about religion every day. I believe in God, and heaven, and purgatory. But not hell. You see, there is something good about everyone, and people need to try harder to find that good. Sometimes I get angry with God, because I have had to deal with mental illness, but I keep trying to understand him. If the Lord loves me, he'll show me a rainbow. I don't go to church, but that doesn't matter, because most people who do are hypocrites."

Energy Information Patterns

Carla, thirty-nine, is a single unemployed transsexual white female living with a male partner. She had a fourteen-year work history in computer programming prior to developing schizophrenia. Carla has a mechanical mind, and her spiritual beliefs, which evolved after the onset of her psychotic disorder, reflect this quality. She says, "The human mind is an energy information pattern that only 'borrows' the brain. Our brains transmit content telepathically, and this content can be stored in the unused portions of other brains up to a radius of several miles away. When we die, our souls, or selves, become linked with other brains, and we can reawaken as spirits. Spirits live within the unused brain material from other people. They travel by moving their energy patterns into brains in new locations. They can tap into a human psychic receiver and send a voice so that you can hear them." Carla states that she became aware of this spirit world when her mind was accidentally rewired to perceive spirit messages and presences. She believes that God exists as an ultimate spirit, perhaps the accumulation of all spirits. "There is no heaven or hell because there is really no end to life." Carla's purpose in living is to understand more about telepathic behavior. She views herself as a scientist. Her partner supports her interests.

The following section introduces concepts that may be helpful to the recovery-oriented practitioner in understanding the spiritual challenges that may accompany the onset and persistence of a mental illness.

The Three Dimensions of Being

As a general framework for attending to a consumer's spiritual concerns, a social worker can attend to the three dimensions of being that are often disrupted by a mental illness. These are being of the world, in the world, and for the world (Frankl, 2000; Lantz, 2002).

The phrase "being of the world" refers to the fact that all people have bodies and must obey the rules of the physical world. This is the *must* dimension of existence. Human beings *must* consume food and water or they will die, *must* die of hypothermia if deprived of clothing and shel-

ter in cold weather, and *must* experience illness if certain biological problems exist within the body. Consumers are in need of medical-oriented
services at times, and thus comprehensive intervention includes the
social worker's willingness to link the consumer to medical providers
when such services are needed. The central intervention issue at the
being of the world dimension of existence is physical vitality.

The term "being in the world" refers to the fact that people have
freedoms and *can* make choices in life reactive to difficulties and opportunities (Berg & Dolan, 2001). All people *can* have an impact on their
inner and outer environments; this is the *can* dimension of existence.
The person has capacities for intentionality and freedom for differentially responding to life situations. A person *can* choose his or her attitude toward life, and in this way manifest "response-ability." It is understood that people from different cultures may view life choices quite
differently. The two central intervention issues at the *can* dimension of
existence are freedom and responsibility.

"Being for the world" refers to the human responsibility to manifest
a self-transcendent style of living in which people answer the call of life
by taking care of other human beings, the community, or the environment. This is the *ought* dimension. People create or discover what they
ought to do in developing a sense of meaning. When a person's sense of
meaning is disrupted, he or she will develop a spiritual vacuum that fills
with either a new sense of meaning or with symptoms such as depression, anxiety, or substance abuse. The two central intervention issues in
the being for the world dimension of existence are meaning and self-
transcendence.

Having broadly considered the importance of spirituality to the
functioning of many recovering consumers—and all people, really—we
can now consider issues more specific to the assessment and intervention processes.

Spiritual Intervention with Recovering Consumers

Again, spiritual issues are not appropriate to address with recovering
consumers in all practice situations (May & Yalom, 2000). In general,
such concerns may not be appropriate for consumers who are absorbed
in immediate problem situations for which they seek practical assistance. On the other hand, purpose-in-life issues may be appropriate for

intervention when the consumer is troubled by anxiety, guilt, and shame, or when he or she demonstrates inclinations to look beyond the self and immediate situation in understanding personal dilemmas. Many recovering consumers seek opportunities to become more complete than they have been (Berg & Dolan, 2001). Spiritual issues should be included to some degree as part of a multidimensional assessment with all consumers, however, because it is always possible that a person's present problems and needs may contribute to, or result from, struggles with broad life concerns.

With regard to utilizing spiritual themes in recovery practice, challenges to social workers are to

- Encourage consumer disclosure of spiritual concerns when appropriate,
- Consider consumer functioning within a broad context of meaning and bring consistency to the consumer's present and ultimate concerns,
- Help consumers identify meanings and purposes that can guide them in making growth-enhancing decisions, and
- Appreciate their own spiritual beliefs and their impact on recovery practice.

Spiritual interventions encourage the consumer to invest actively in constructive life activity, to look externally for solutions to problems rather than be preoccupied with internal emotions, and to care about something outside the self.

Assessment

A variety of instruments have been developed to assist with a social worker's spiritual assessments, but informal questioning can work just as well. Five strategies are presented here. The first of these (adapted from Sheridan, 2008) is the most detailed, and includes the following questions:

- Do you consider yourself to be a spiritual person? What does the word "spiritual" mean to you?
- What nourishes you spiritually? For example, music, nature, relationships, meditation, creative expression, sharing another's joy?

- Do you believe there is a Supreme Being? If so, what does that being look like?
- What were some of the important faith or spiritual issues in your family background?
- Was there ever an incident in your life that precipitated a change in your belief about the meaning of life?
- How and when have you prayed or meditated? What is the difference?
- What is your opinion about the meaning of suffering?

Many of the above questions are directly religious in nature, and some social workers may thus be uncomfortable with asking them. The next questioning route is broader, and organizes the spiritual assessment along seven dimensions (Koenig & Pritchett, 1998):

1. Beliefs and meanings: how the person develops a sense of purpose
2. Vocations and consequences: how the person understands his or her obligations and the consequences of meeting or not meeting them
3. Experience and emotion: the affective tone of spiritual life
4. Courage and growth: how the consumer faces challenges and doubts
5. Rituals and practice: how the person enacts key beliefs
6. Participation in a religious or spiritual community
7. Where the person locates authority and guidance for his or her core beliefs

This approach to assessment offers several advantages. Its conception of spirituality is intentionally broad, so it is useful in settings where diverse religious cultures exist. Furthermore, since it assumes that all people have a spiritual dimension, it can be helpful whether or not the consumer identifies him- or herself as spiritual.

An adaptation of the above strategy (Fallott, 1998) attends to only four of a consumer's spiritual domains (beliefs and meaning, experience and emotion, rituals and practice, and community) and explores the following three related questions:

1. How explicitly does the consumer use religious language to express experiences in each domain?

2. What is the positive or negative role of each domain in the recovery process?
3. How might spirituality be included in the service plan?

Another, even simpler, format for spiritual assessment proposes a consideration of only four questions (Koenig & Pritchett, 1998):

1. Is religious faith an important part of your life?
2. How has your faith influenced your life, past and present?
3. Are you part of a religious or spiritual community?
4. Are there any spiritual needs that you would like me to address in our work together?

Regardless of its degree of structure, a spiritual assessment has considerable value in recovery practice. Asking about these issues communicates the social worker's interest in more than a symptom-oriented evaluation and facilitates the exploration of an area of potential significance to the consumer's recovery. We now turn to the process of utilizing these issues in practice.

Individual Intervention

Although it is important for the spiritual practitioner to have a firmly developed knowledge base and intervention framework, the specific nature of the spiritual elements of that work is always unique to the characteristics of each consumer (Lantz & Gregoire, 2000). In this context, spiritual pain can be defined as a consumer's negative emotional reaction to the occurrence of a stressful and difficult event related to his or her sense of purpose in life (Lantz, 1978; Walsh, 2007). A healing process occurs when the practitioner helps the consumer to hold the pain leading to spiritual dilemmas, tell the pain, master the pain, and honor the pain (Lantz, 2002). This process, which need not be separate from other interventions the social worker is providing, is described below, with an example.

Holding the Pain   People often push significant challenges out of their awareness to avoid the experience of pain. In spiritual intervention, the word "holding" refers to a process of holding up the challenge (often isolation and estrangement) so it may be seen by the consumer. Holding up the problem includes reexperiencing the pain at its core, but it also includes catharsis. As a consumer holds up and reexperiences negative feelings, he or she often releases pain and so reduces suffering.

Holding is sometimes described as empathic availability, or a committed presence to the other and openness to the pain of the other. When manifesting empathic availability, the social worker does not hide from the consumer's spiritual distress behind a stance of objectivity. The social worker must persist with a well-formulated intervention stance, but such a concern should not result in blunted compassion. Empathic availability provides the consumer with the support needed to help him or her tell the story of the spiritual challenge. The practitioner's empathic availability and willingness to share the consumer's pain allows the consumer to reexperience that pain without defensiveness.

Sarah's Torment

Sarah was a thirty-four-year-old single Jewish woman, living alone in an apartment complex, with a history of schizophrenia. She had been actively psychotic since late adolescence, hearing the voices of various Biblical figures and of God, which sometimes tormented her for being a bad person, and sometimes soothed her. Furthermore, she believed she was the reincarnation of Anne Frank, the young diarist who was killed by the Nazis. Sarah's two parents, with whom she had conflicted relationships, lived five hundred miles away and served as her payees, and she was estranged from her two brothers. She led a lonely, isolated life and dwelled frequently on her religious beliefs and culture. Sarah was convinced that she was suffering with mental illness, and was being tested by God so that the Jewish people in general could flourish. Her social worker, who was an atheist, became aware of her religious preoccupations early in their relationship. Sarah at first was uncomfortable raising these issues because her family had always discouraged her from doing so. The social worker encouraged Sarah to share her ideas, however, because they were so important to her. He listened and affirmed that Sarah was doing her best to understand what her calling in life might be. At the beginning of most of their sessions, Sarah described her latest experiences with God and suffering, and she clearly felt a great sense of relief and validation in doing so. The social worker never commented on the reality of her thoughts.

Telling the Pain   Telling, talking about, and naming emotional pain is the second element of spiritual intervention. Such telling places the emotional experience into the world of mutual encounter, where the relationship can be used to process the consumer's concerns under circumstances of increased support. Telling emotional experience brings pain out of the internal world of the consumer and into the interactional world of mutual awareness, understanding, and support. A second reason why telling the pain is helpful has to do with the power of naming. When a consumer can describe, tell, and name the experienced emotions, he or she begins the process of mastering it.

Sarah's Torment (cont.)

The social worker encouraged Sarah to speak with a rabbi about her experiences, but Sarah did not want to do so, saying that in the past she had not been taken seriously. The social worker was sometimes uncomfortable hearing about Sarah's religious experiences, because he did not believe they were objectively true and he understood that they interfered with her ability to manage everyday relationships and activities of daily living. He was, however, able to help Sarah understand that her ideas reflected her desire to make a contribution to other members of the Jewish faith. Sarah did understand that she had a mental illness, but she was never sure which elements of her experiences were real and which were not. While exploring her ideas, Sarah expressed a firm belief that she had an important role in taking care of her parents, because, in her words, she was "absorbing" their own pain and sending out "healing warmth" toward them. During their conversations, Sarah thus developed a constructive rationale for why she had to live as she did, framing it as being for the benefit of others. Again, the social worker did not agree with these ideas, but he could see that Sarah's processing of them had helped her develop a more affirming understanding of herself.

It should be emphasized that the social worker was providing Sarah with other interventions during this process. He was, for example, coordinating appointments with the psychiatrist for Sarah's regular medication evaluations, about which she was compliant, and helping her problem solve with regard to basic responsibilities related to budgeting and home care.

Mastering the Pain   Mastering the pain is a process of behavioral experimentation that helps a consumer find unique healing activities that are useful in processing concerns and moving toward spiritual growth. From a spiritual point of view, helping a consumer transform aggression into assertiveness, avoidance into independence, and dependence into the ability to experience deeper connections is a powerful way to master his or her emotional experiences. Mastering the pain helps a consumer develop freedom at the "being of the world" dimension of existence, which includes noticing meaning potentials or, in other words, taking advantage of a growth opportunity.

Sarah's Torment (cont.)

The social worker tried to help Sarah's recovery in many ways, including considering how she might be less isolated and lonely. The client wanted to have more of a social life and also begin working again; in the past she had worked as a receptionist in several small businesses. Still, she had a limited tolerance for interaction with others. She was also a college graduate with an English degree who loved to read, and she wanted to join a book club. Sarah did not wish, however, to participate in consumer-run activities, because she felt, as she put it, "more normal" than other people with mental illness. Given Sarah's interest in spirituality, the social worker encouraged her to seek out volunteer opportunities at a local synagogue as one way of taking a possibly comfortable step into a social milieu. She might, for example, be able to drive elderly persons to religious events and so provide an important service while maintaining limited exposure to others. This idea was appealing to Sarah.

Honoring the Pain   Honoring the pain is a process of celebrating the meaning potentials and opportunities in the problem situation. It involves the consumer's becoming aware of opportunities for self-transcendent giving to the world that are embedded in the problem situation. During the process of honoring the pain, the practitioner helps the consumer develop greater self-understanding and perhaps find ways to contribute to the lives of others, if the consumer is inclined to do so. This helps the consumer to manifest existence at the "being for the world" dimension. Honoring is a celebration of the mastering of one's emotional pain, and is a way to fill the spiritual meaning vacuum that often occurs reactive to a traumatic experience.

Sarah's Torment (cont.)

Sarah did not move far into this level, although she made some progress. As a result of her reflections with the social worker, she decided to stay in direct contact with her parents more often to check on their well-being and to express openly that she cared for them. The social worker encouraged Sarah to think more broadly about how her existence could be a positive element in the lives of others by becoming active in help-giving activities that did not pertain strictly to her religious preoccupations. Sarah decided that she would try harder to be friendly with other people in her apartment complex and participate more in that community. She could honor the fact that she was suffering on behalf of others by making small contributions to the lives of more people, and by being a good neighbor. This seemed like a reasonable idea to her social worker, although he planned to monitor Sarah's activities carefully so that she was not mocked or taken advantage of by others.

The social worker was involved in Sarah's life for two years. She experienced many setbacks and several hospitalizations due to the severity of her disorder during that period. His attention to her spiritual preoccupations was generally helpful in the consumer's ability to add variety to her activities of daily living, and to think more broadly about the role of religion in her life, but she did not make major progress in reducing her overall symptoms.

For consumers who are interested in developing their spiritual natures through education and discussion, various group intervention formats are available. What follows are descriptions of three groups that have been utilized toward this end. None of these has been extensively evaluated for effectiveness, so it must be emphasized that they are only examples of possibilities for group intervention.

Group Interventions

The Spiritual Beliefs and Values Group   The Spiritual Beliefs and Values Group is an open-ended psychodynamic group that provides consumers with a forum to examine and explore their religious beliefs and spiritual concerns (Kehoe, 1998). The leader, who has conducted the group for sixteen years, does not provide didactic content but instead allows the members to use the time in ways that are most important to them. The leader's task is to facilitate discussion in which consumers can make connections between their ideas about spirituality and its relationship to their current lives. Among the positive elements of the group are members' improved capacities for relating their beliefs to everyday life situations and for discovering their common search for meaning and purpose; the evaluation is based on consumer feedback.

The Spirituality Psychoeducation Group   Two other groups of this type are more structured. The first is a four-session, ninety-minute psychodynamic group that addresses how one's spiritual beliefs can enhance self-esteem and self-worth (Lindgren & Coursey, 1995). This model offers an appealing format to consumers who prefer a time-limited experience. The following four topics are included in the series:

1. Self-esteem, spirituality, and their relationship to social values
2. Spiritual meanings connected to one's mental disorder, and their implications for the consumer's sense of self-worth
3. Forgiving one's failures, celebrating successes, and recognizing personal qualities that members can offer to the lives of others
4. The impact of spiritual experiences and social support on one's functioning

This intervention was evaluated using thirty consumers who were interested in addressing their spirituality, drawn from three psychosocial rehabilitation centers in one city. Six groups were conducted and used in the evaluation. Data were presented on the participants' religious service attendance, use of prayer and religious thoughts, discussions of spirituality in therapy, the effects of spirituality on their illness and lives, and unusual spiritual experiences. Significant pre- and post-changes on most measures were found through the use of a spiritual support scale, but not on measures of depression, hopelessness, self-esteem, or perceived purpose in life.

The Spirituality and Trauma Recovery Group   Another intervention alternative is a nine-session spirituality group that includes specific topics and goals that, while structured, is less didactic than traditional psychoeducational programs (Fallot & Newburn, 2000). The purposes of the program are to help members deal with their spiritual struggles as well as to identify spiritual resources for their recovery. The program is organized as follows:

- Three sessions are devoted to reflecting on and discussing consumers' spiritual histories, related positive resources, and coping strategies.
- Three sessions focus on consumers' experiences that lead to spiritual struggles and call for a response; such experiences commonly feature fear and powerlessness, anger and resentment, and despair and hopelessness.
- Three final sessions are devoted to facing the future, including hope, vision, and continuing the journey of healing.

Each session is built around a set of questions and an exercise designed to clarify ways in which members may utilize group content in their spiritual lives.

Environmental Interventions

Recovery practice always involves the social worker's helping consumers take advantage of available community supports. Social workers can support consumers' inclinations for spiritual fellowship in this way by being aware of, and making referrals to, religious organizations and other related community resources. This may be a preferable form of intervention for practitioners who do not feel comfortable dealing with a consumer's spiritual concerns and who believe that other persons (pastors, rabbis, etc.) are more appropriate for the task. Toward this end, social workers should nurture relationships with area faith communities and other sources of spiritual support. Recovery practitioners should develop knowledge about all possible sources of spiritual support, not just, for example, the locations and times of major religious services. Developing this knowledge demands that social workers be willing to collaborate with religious professionals or healers in arranging for consumer support when indicated; to address in intervention plans, when appropriate, goals for helping consumers find a responsive spiritual community; and to participate in professional development to enhance consumers' awareness of religious and spiritual organizations in their areas of practice.

Faith communities and other spiritual resources may offer many consumers a sense of belonging, shared meaning, tangible and emotional support, and structure that gives purpose to their lives. It must be emphasized, however, that some religious organizations (or members of those organizations) may in fact reject persons who are struggling with mental illness. As an example, one of the author's consumers, after sharing his experience with past physical abuse and depression in a church discussion group, was told by another member, "Depression is no reason to stay in bed; that is just Satan."

Summary

Secular and nonsecular conceptions of spirituality represent important, basic concerns to most people, with implications for how they find meaning and purpose and develop values that give direction to their lives. With the onset and persistence of mental illness, consumers may face major challenges to their spiritual value systems. They experience disruptions to their sense of self and as such often dwell openly on concerns related to purpose and meaning in life. Attention to consumers' spiritual concerns is thus important to recovery-oriented social workers. Spiritual issues may not be appropriate to address with consumers in all practice situations, however, especially when they are absorbed in problem situations for which they seek immediate and concrete assistance. On the other hand, purpose-in-life issues may be appropriate for intervention when the consumer demonstrates inclinations to look beyond the self and immediate situation in understanding personal dilemmas.

Many social workers and other human services practitioners are uncomfortable with addressing issues of spirituality with recovering consumers, especially when those issues involve ideas that appear to be related to psychosis. The recent movement away from depth psychology toward a (supposedly) more scientific and quantifiable orientation to practice puts some approaches to social work at a disadvantage in addressing these issues. Despite this trend, recovery practitioners need to recognize the importance of spirituality in their work. They should be respectful of different religious or spiritual paths, and be willing to learn about the role and meaning of the beliefs, practices, and experiences of various types of consumers. They should be informed about the positive and negative roles of religion and spirituality among members of oppressed poulations. Finally, social workers should develop a working knowledge of the beliefs and practices frequently encountered in their practice, and engage in ongoing self-reflection about what brings purpose and meaning to their own lives.

Major Chapter Learning Points

- Spirituality can be broadly defined as one's search for and adherence to ultimate meanings, purposes, and commitments in life.
- Spirituality may be evident in a person's belief systems, social concerns, creative pursuits, and sense of hope for a better future.
- Three dimensions of being that are often disrupted by a mental illness, and that may be targeted for spiritual intervention, are being of the world, in the world, and for the world.
- A spiritual assessment communicates the social worker's interest in more than a symptom-oriented evaluation, and facilitates the exploration of an area of potential significance to the consumer's recovery.
- One framework for providing spiritually focused interventions for individuals is to help the consumer hold the pain, tell the pain, master the pain, and honor the pain.
- Several group interventions are available for addressing the spiritual concerns of recovering consumers.
- Developing competence for addressing a consumer's spiritual needs demands that social workers be willing to collaborate with religious professionals or healers in arranging for consumer support, and be willing to help consumers locate a responsive spiritual community.

Questions for Reflection or Discussion

1. Reflect on your own spirituality, however you experience it, and consider how it might be a benefit and a limitation in your work with recovering consumers. Would you feel comfortable talking with a supervisor about these issues? Why or why not?

2. To what extent would you feel comfortable addressing specifically religious (doctrinal) issues with consumers? Develop some hypothetical examples and consider how you might respond to them.

3. Think about ways in which spirituality can be a negative force in consumers' lives, and how you might address those negatives when they appear.

4. Do you think that the will to meaning, and the three dimensions of being, as discussed in this chapter, are useful frameworks for conceiving of a consumer's spirituality? Are you aware of other frameworks?

Part 2

Recovery
Interventions
for Specific
Mental
Disorders

Chapter 7

Schizophrenia

Schizophrenia is a mental disorder characterized by a person's abnormal patterns of thought and perception. It includes two types of symptoms (APA, 2000): (1) Positive symptoms represent exaggerations of normal behavior and include hallucinations, delusions, disorganized thinking, and tendencies toward agitation. (2) Negative symptoms represent the absence of what would be considered normal behavior and include flat affect (the absence of expression), social withdrawal, noncommunication, passivity, and ambivalence in decision making. Schizophrenia is considered to be a chronic disorder, one in which the symptoms wax and wane over the course of one's life. It has a worldwide prevalence of approximately 1 percent (Murray, Jones, & Susser, 2003).

As noted in chapter 2, the emergence of research-based knowledge about the wide variability in outcomes for persons with schizophrenia was a major force behind the emergence of the recovery movement. What was once considered a disorder with an unremitting downward course was found to have encouraging outcomes as well. Social workers have learned to carry few assumptions about the prognosis for persons with the diagnosis. This chapter begins with information about risk and resilience factors significant to the onset and course of schizophrenia, and then considers two lengthy case illustrations of recovery-based practice by social workers.

Risk and Resilience Influences for Onset

The specific causes of schizophrenia are not known. The stress or diathesis theory holds that schizophrenia results from a mix of heritability and biological influences (perhaps 70 percent) and environmental and stress factors (approximately 30 percent) (Cardno & Murray, 2003), which may include brain injury and threatening physical environments.

Biological Influences

Biological theories of schizophrenia implicate the brain's limbic system (center of emotional activity), frontal cortex (governing personality, emotion, and reasoning), and basal ganglia (regulating muscle and skeletal movement) as primary sites of malfunction (Conklin & Iacono, 2003). People with schizophrenia are believed to have a relatively high concentration of the neurotransmitter dopamine in nerve cell pathways extending into the cortex and limbic system. Other neurotransmitters, including serotonin and norepinephrine, have also been proposed as risk influences (van Os, Rutten, Bart, & Poulton, 2008). Some researchers are studying the influences of certain chromosomes on molecular pathways in the brain as causal mechanisms for schizophrenia (Detera-Wadleigh & McMahon, 2006), but this work remains speculative. Still, its genetic transmission is supported by the higher-than-average risk among family members of persons with the disorder (Ivleva, Thaker, & Tamminga, 2008).

Psychosocial Influences

There are no known psychological influences of specific stress events on the development of schizophrenia, although many years ago events such as emotional deprivation, stunted psychosocial development, and erratic parenting were considered to be dominant causes (Phillips, Francey, Edwards, & McMurray, 2007). There are, however, some social risk influences for schizophrenia. These stresses include living in an urban environment, being born into relatively low socioeconomic status, and migrating into a new culture (Selten, Cantor-Craae, & Kahn, 2007). Conversely, living in a rural environment, being of middle- or upper-class socioeconomic status, and geographic stability are protective influences.

Risk and Resilience Influences for Course

Major factors influencing the course of schizophrenia can be summarized as follows:

- Gradual onset (protective) versus sudden or later onset of symptoms (risk)
- Relative absence versus prominence of negative symptoms

- Good versus poor interepisode functioning
- Insight versus lack of insight into the disorder
- Presence versus absence of social skills
- Stress-free versus stressful family environment
- Presence versus absence of a support system
- Living in a rural versus urban area
- Moderate amount of social stimulation versus too little or too much
- Attitudes of acceptance versus rejection or avoidance from others
- Reasonable versus excessive or no expectations from others
- The opportunity to develop and practice vocational skills

While recovery practices need not be limited to the professionally developed interventions for persons with schizophrenia, it is important to describe what is known about those practices.

Standard Interventions

There is a consensus that intervention for schizophrenia should be multimodal and include strategies targeted at both specific symptoms and the social and educational needs of the consumer and his or her family (Spaulding & Nolting, 2006). One literature review established that consumer satisfaction with interventions for schizophrenia is influenced by multiple factors, including an absence of significant medication side effects, participation in treatment planning, and participation of family members and significant others (Chue, 2006).

Medications

Medication is a primary intervention modality for persons with schizophrenia. It cannot cure a person of the disorder, but it can eliminate or reduce some of the symptoms. Almost all physicians recommend antipsychotic medication for persons with schizophrenia, but their relative risks and benefits with regard to the consumer's physical and emotional well-being are subject to debate (Cohen, 2002). Studies of drug effectiveness for the symptoms of schizophrenia consistently indicate that many consumers discontinue their medication for a variety of reasons, such as perceived ineffectiveness and adverse effects (Lieberman et al., 2005). The significance of adverse effects on a consumer's physical, as well as psychological and social, well-being cannot be overstated (Bentley & Walsh, 2006). The newer medications have less adverse effects overall, but they are not devoid of them, as will be demonstrated later in this chapter, in the intervention vignettes.

Psychosocial Interventions

Research on psychodynamic interventions for schizophrenia provides limited empirical support (Malmberg & Fenton, 2005). One positive aspect of this type of intervention, however, is that it alerts the practitioner to the importance of the social worker–consumer relationship, as detailed in chapter 5.

Cognitive-behavioral therapy (CBT) is increasingly being used to help persons with schizophrenia (Kuipers, Garety, & Fowler, 2006). CBT interventions are based on the premise that current beliefs and attitudes mediate a person's moods and behaviors to a significant extent. CBT focuses on a review of the consumer's core beliefs regarding self-worth, the ability to create changes in his or her life, and the establishment of realistic goals. Consumers are helped to modify their assumptions about the self, the world, and the future; improve coping responses to stressful events and life challenges; relabel some psychotic experiences as symptoms rather than external reality; and improve their social skills.

Group interventions include insight-oriented, supportive, and behavioral modalities. For persons with schizophrenia, groups focused on increased social interaction and learning about and managing symptoms are often effective (Kanas, 2005). A systematic review of five controlled trials of group CBT for schizophrenia indicated that benefits were also evident with regard to some symptoms, most prominently anxiety and depression (Lawrence, Bradshaw, & Mairs, 2006).

Family participation in a consumer's intervention is a protective influence (Pharoah, Rathbone, Mari, & Streiner, 2003). When a person has schizophrenia, a chronic emotional burden develops that is shared by all family members. Their common reactions include stress, anxiety, resentment of the impaired member, grief, and depression. Family interventions in schizophrenia usually focus in part on producing a more positive atmosphere for all members, which in turn contributes to the consumer's positive adjustment.

Case management refers to a variety of community-based intervention modalities designed to help consumers receive a full range of
support and rehabilitation services in a timely, appropriate fashion
(Northway, 2005). Practitioners attend to relevant issues in the consumer's family, neighborhood, and community, and focus on medical
health, employment, income, housing, and social support. These interventions are often carried out in the context of large, community-based
programs. The core characteristics include assertive engagement, service delivery in the consumer's natural environment, a multidiscipli-
nary team approach, staff continuity over time, low staff-to-consumer
ratios, and frequent consumer contacts. Services are provided in the
consumer's home or wherever the consumer feels comfortable, and
focus on everyday needs. Frequency of contact is variable, depending
on assessed consumer need. Recovery-focused interventions are often
provided in the context of these teams.

The remainder of this chapter includes extended examples of
recovery-oriented social work practice with two consumers, both of
whom are diagnosed with schizoaffective disorder, a disorder that features the symptoms of schizophrenia along with a significant range of
emotional experiences. In each of these situations, the consumer does
not overtly acknowledge that he or she has a disorder, but nevertheless
chooses, initially with some reluctance, to work with a social worker.
The practitioners in these cases rely in part on the formal intervention
strategies described above but mainly focus on their relationship-
building capacities to engage the consumer in a self-directed recovery
process. This focus, in fact, is what distinguishes their recovery orientation. Each illustration will primarily demonstrate the recovery interventions described in chapter 4 of engagement, sustainment and processing distress, expanding the consumer's perspective, facilitating new
understandings, and introducing new possibilities for action.

The Angry Attorney

Kyle was an experienced social worker in a comprehensive
community services agency. A law permitting the outpatient
commitment of persons with serious mental illness had recently
been passed in Kyle's state. For the first time, persons judged to
be dangerous to self or others due to a mental illness could be

committed to a community mental health center instead of a hospital. The rationale behind this law was that these consumers would be permitted to function in the least restrictive environment as long as they complied with outpatient intervention. If the consumer did not follow through with such intervention, he or she could be involuntarily placed in a psychiatric hospital for the remainder of the probationary period.

Jacqui Thomas was one of the first persons in the state to receive an outpatient commitment. Her parents had committed her for ninety days to a state hospital following a psychotic break, but forty-five days into her hospital stay she was released without a change in legal status. The hospital staff assessed that Jacqui had sufficiently stabilized that she did not require further hospitalization. She was referred to Kyle's community mental health center with the county MHA's approval.

Jacqui was a forty-year-old divorced Lebanese American woman with degrees in law and taxation who carried a diagnosis of schizoaffective disorder. She met criteria for schizophrenia, but also displayed a full range of mood functioning, often becoming alternately agitated or depressed. Jacqui had been practicing law in the Middle East for the past year when her family was summoned to come and get her. She had become paranoid and agitated, publicly accusing governments from several nations of conspiring against her well-being because of her rising leadership in the legal community. Jacqui had been calling and berating government officials and her legal opponents for supposed defamatory activities against her, and in so doing had lost her job and ruined her legal reputation in that area. Her family took Jacqui back to their home in the Midwest and then to the hospital after a series of confrontations with neighbors and police officers. Jacqui was wildly upset about these developments, seeing them as part of a larger conspiracy against her. Among other things, she came to believe that her younger sister, who had died of cancer six years ago at the age of twenty-seven, had been murdered by the United States government as a warning against Jacqui's legal advocacy stances. When admitted to the state facility, Jacqui was forcibly given injectible antipsychotic medications, which calmed her moderately but generated strong adverse effects of muscle stiffness. Jacqui believed that she was a political prisoner.

Jacqui was the second of four daughters born to her Lebanese parents Michael (now seventy-five) and Rachel (seventy-two). They had been a close-knit family, and the children were brought up to view their ethnic values as superior to, and often in conflict with, mainstream American society. All four girls were taught by their parents to stick together and distrust the motives of others, who were likely to have prejudices against them. Michael had been a laborer all his life, holding a variety of jobs while establishing a minimally secure income base.

The daughters were raised to be high-achievers and to make the family proud of them. Rita (forty-two), the oldest daughter, had aspired to be an interior decorator but had floundered in her business ventures. She was married and divorced with an eight-year-old daughter. Rebecca, age thirty-eight, was married with two children and lived far away from the family, and had only occasional contact with them. The youngest daughter, Terri, had tragically died. Jacqui had always been the best of the best in her family's eyes, and was encouraged to pursue her academic interests. Jacqui had married at age twenty-five but had been divorced for ten years at the time of this episode. She had one previous major psychotic break, similar to the present one, at age thirty-three, and had taken medication for several years afterward before terminating that intervention. At this time, Jacqui believed that nothing was wrong with her, and that all of her perceptions were accurate.

Engagement

Kyle's initial meeting with Jacqui, excerpted here, was dramatic. Her sister Rita, who appeared to be taking charge in the delicate situation, accompanied Jacqui to the session. Rita was friendly, impeccably groomed, articulate, and prone to lecturing Jacqui that she needed to cooperate. Jacqui was angry and not in a cooperative mood. She could not sit or stand still, and her arms shook throughout the forty-five-minute session due to adverse effects of the medication.

She said to Kyle, a thirty-eight-year-old Caucasian male, "They say I have to come here until you say I don't have to. So if you want to help me, do that! Write a letter to the governor saying I don't need to be here."

Kyle was experienced in working with consumers who had severe mental illnesses. He was calm, pleasant, and honest. "I can't do that right now, Jacqui. I've just met you. The MHA will want reasons for whatever I say, and I can't give them anything right now."

"So you're useless. You can't help me at all. There's nothing wrong with me. I don't want you or anyone else here messing with me. I'm not taking medicine, that's for sure. If you try to make me do anything against my will, I swear I'll sue you." Jacqui was screaming, and other staff in the small agency could hear their exchange. Rita repeatedly tried to calm her sister, but Kyle kept his focus on Jacqui.

Kyle was a recovery-focused social worker, accustomed to working cooperatively with consumers, so he offered a compromise. "I tell you what, Jacqui. I know you think the commitment is unfair, and you don't want to do anything against your will. One thing's for sure, and I say this based on my knowledge of the mental health system: your commitment is likely to go beyond ninety days if you completely refuse to participate with us. You need to understand that. I suggest that you agree to be involved with the agency, and with me, to some extent for the next forty-five days. I won't expect anything from you other than minimal participation. That way I can get to know you and later write a more informed letter to the MHA."

"I don't like the sound of that. What will we do?"

Kyle believed that Jacqui might benefit from formal intervention, but he always respected his consumers' wishes, and tried to see the world through their eyes. "We don't have to do anything other than meet occasionally for an hour or so. Of course, we'll be spending time together, so hopefully we can talk, but as far as what we talk about, it would be up to you."

"How often will we have to meet?"

"Do you have a suggestion?"

Jacqui was quick with her response. "Yes, I think we should meet monthly. That way I'll see you maybe two more times, and I'll be in compliance, and you can write a letter saying I should be released. How about that?"

Kyle gave an honest response. "It's true that some people only come here once per month, but that's because they've been coming for a while, and we know them, and all they're doing is checking in with the doctor or social worker. I really don't think the MHA would be okay with two total visits. How about every other week? And I'll tell you what: to make it more convenient for you, Jacqui, we can trade off making the trip. We can alternate meeting here and at your home, if that's okay with you and your family."

Jacqui was unenthusiastic but agreed to the idea. "I guess that'll be okay. But I still don't know what we'll do when we meet. You'd better not try to talk me into anything! Like I said, I'll sue you, and you'll lose your license."

"I hear you, Jacqui." There was another topic that Kyle needed to raise. "Now, there's something else to talk about here. You've been taking medication, right? Our physician should check with you about those, now that you're out of the hospital."

Jacqui began shouting again. "Absolutely not! I'm not seeing a doctor! I'm not taking medications! They've been shooting me up at the hospital and look at me! The government is trying to incapacitate me, and it's working!"

Kyle was sympathetic. "I'm not saying you have to keep taking medication, Jacqui. That's not my call anyway. I'm saying you should check in with the doctor here, because you're on medication now, and it would irresponsible of him not to follow up. I can see that you're stiff and shaking, and I know you hate that. Look, I know Dr. Morris very well. [He and Kyle had worked together for five years.] I'll talk with him about your situation, and I'll introduce you to him, and I'll make sure he knows you don't want to be on meds. I don't know what he'll say about that. But it's your right to make that decision. No one here will force medications on you." From what Kyle knew about Jacqui's history and presenting situation, he hoped she would decide to take medications.

"And all of this will get me off probation?"

"I can't guarantee anything, Jacqui. It's not my ultimate decision to make. You understand that, according to the law, the MHA psychiatrists and attorneys will make that decision. The doctor and I will be asked for our opinions, though, and I promise to report the truth about your participation here, and I'll tell you in advance what we're going to write." Kyle was quite aware that any serious symptomatic problems that might develop could result in Jacqui's return to the hospital.

The meeting ended with this point of agreement, although Jacqui's sister told her, "It'll be best if you take medicine and get counselling from Kyle. You know that." The sisters started arguing again, and in the midst of their raised voices Kyle scheduled another appointment with the consumer.

Kyle did not intend his interactions with Jacqui to be manipulative. He was genuinely trying to accommodate her perspectives. Kyle believed that Jacqui had a mental disorder, and that her judgment was impaired at this time, although he had not been able to complete a full assessment based on that first meeting and the hospital records. He thought Jacqui might be more likely to have a satisfying life if she accepted a range of medication and psychosocial interventions from the agency. Still, Kyle was not going to go against her will. He believed that if he could engage Jacqui in a cooperative relationship in accordance with her goals, initially limited to "getting off probation," she might see that she had power in the intervention process and decide to accept his assistance. They agreed to meet again at her home in two weeks, and that she would come back to the agency to meet the physician one week after the home visit, when the effects of her medication would be wearing off.

Kyle accepted Jacqui's formal diagnosis of schizoaffective disorder as accurate, but he did not base his ideas for intervention on it. He was more attuned to his consumer's motivations. Jacqui had considerable strengths, including intelligence; competence, with several graduate degrees and a law practice focused on minority consumers; and a history of good interpersonal relations. She also demonstrated a strong sense of purpose, of being for the world, in her legal advocacy activities on behalf of the Lebanese community. Still, at this time she felt alienated from almost everyone. She was convinced that most other people were her intellectual inferiors, pawns in government conspiracies against her.

Jacqui's perception of her situation was one of forced compliance with an unjust legal mandate. She expected Kyle to try to convince her of the need for treatment, as professional staff at the hospital had done. The issue of unequal power was a major constraint to her potential for developing a cooperative relationship with a social worker. It required that she subject herself to the will of the social worker and agency. Given Jacqui's perspectives, Kyle agreed to meet her where she was and attempt to show her that they could share power, and that he might become a partner in her desire to end her probation. There was certainly nothing to be gained by confronting her negative attitudes, but beyond that Kyle respected her position. There was no telling at this point how Jacqui's thoughts and feelings would evolve during the coming weeks, or how her symptoms might fluctuate. Kyle believed that he could focus on the recovery principles of relationship development and consistent application of recovery values in which interventions are based on the consumer's preferences.

Sustainment and Processing Distress

Because of scheduling complications at the agency, Kyle and Jacqui met twice more before the physician's appointment. Their next visit was at Jacqui's apartment, which pleased the consumer because it gave her a sense of power over the interaction and distance from the agency, where she felt stigmatized. Kyle noticed a major change in Jacqui's affect during this visit. She was showing fewer signs of muscle stiffness, seemed more relaxed, and was much better groomed. She looked ten years younger, and had a pleasant, though rare, smile.

Jacqui didn't want to let Kyle inside, and since it was a nice day they sat on the front porch. The consumer immediately challenged him. "So what are we supposed to do today? How long do you have to stay? Don't expect me to tell you much. There's nothing wrong with me."

Kyle was prepared, and responded, "I know you don't like this, Jacqui, but we agreed to this plan. Like I said, I don't know what we'll do today. I hope we can talk, and maybe get to know each other, but I have no agenda." When Jacqui said that they might as well stop the visit right then, Kyle said, "For example, Jacqui, I know you've done a lot of interesting work as an attorney, and that you've traveled a lot. Can you tell me about your work? I haven't traveled much. I'd like to hear about that."

Jacqui seemed surprised. "I guess so, but don't try to get personal. And you'd better not be trying to set me up to look bad."

They talked socially for an hour. Kyle was genuinely interested in Jacqui's travels and work history. He learned that she had published a few articles in law journals and headed a regional bar association in Europe. Jacqui warmed up to Kyle's easygoing, inquisitive manner and became more enthusiastic as they talked. At one point she actually laughed, and said, "I must say, I'm enjoying this." Later, though, she repeated, "I still don't know what to make of you, and what you're up to. The only thing you could do to really help me would be to help get my law license back. All I want is to be an attorney. You have no power in that area." Kyle agreed, but said, "Maybe I can help you have a better chance of getting your license back. Maybe I can help these next six weeks go by smoothly so you have more control over your life than you do now." Jacqui agreed to set as her goal "to get my law license back," but she would not write that down or agree to any particular steps toward that end. Still, this was her vision, and her ultimate goal.

During these weeks, Kyle had occasional phone contact with Jacqui's sister Rita and her mother Rachel. Jacqui had permitted these contacts on the condition that Kyle let her know when any family members called him. These calls were helpful in that they helped Kyle monitor Jacqui's moods and behavior. It seemed that she was staying close to home, quietly helping to keep up the apartment and watching her young niece. Still, Jacqui often talked with the family about feeling victimized by government agents, and they were justifiably concerned about her. It was usually Rita who called Kyle and asked that he "do something" about her sister's strange thinking by "getting her to take more medicine." Kyle listened sympathetically, and got along well with the family, but defended his position of working with Jacqui on her stated goals at her own pace. He invited Jacqui's parents and sister to attend a family education and support group being conducted at his agency, and Rachel accepted the offer, becoming a regular member of the nine-session group. This was a psychoeducational group in which family members learned about the nature of schizophrenia and its interventions; much time was reserved each week for members to process their concerns about their recovering relatives.

Two weeks later, Jacqui and Kyle met at the agency and had another pleasant conversation. Jacqui was enjoying Kyle's company. She seemed to be developing trust in the social worker and no longer warned him of possible lawsuits if he betrayed her in any way. Understanding Jacqui's negative attitude about the agency, the worker continued to encourage her to ventilate her feelings about her prior incarceration and current outpatient commitment. Jacqui was calming down and began to value the relationship even as she continued to discount her need for services. She seemed to perceive Kyle as the one person she might be able to trust. One difference in the structure of this visit is that Kyle needed to talk with Jacqui about the upcoming physician's appointment. Jacqui's resolve stiffened again. "I'm not taking meds. I'll see the doctor, but I'm not taking meds. If you want to help me, make that happen."

As he had promised, Kyle met with the physician in advance of their appointment and explained Jacqui's situation. The two men had an excellent working relationship, and Dr. Morris agreed to do no more than encourage the consumer to take medication if he believed that she might benefit from them. Kyle decided not to attend the meeting so as not to become involved in any possible disagreements that might arise. Dr. Morris agreed that his presence would encourage Jacqui to see Kyle as her advocate. He escorted Jacqui to the meeting, introduced her to the physician, and left. Dr. Morris had a pleasant and nonthreatening interpersonal style, and Jacqui later said that she felt respected during their thirty-minute meeting. She agreed to meet with the physician every two weeks, even though she refused his recommendation of medications. Dr. Morris wanted to monitor her mental status and Jacqui viewed this (correctly) as a strategy that would keep her in compliance with the dictates of the probation board.

Jacqui was pleased with this agreement, but her mother and sister were upset to learn that she would not be taking medications. They called and pleaded with the social worker to "talk Jacqui into" taking the medicine. Kyle did not agree to this, but assured the family that both he and Dr. Morris would closely monitor the situation, and that they could continue to call if they had concerns.

During subsequent meetings, the social worker invited Jacqui to talk more specifically about some of her career frustrations and how she might try to work them out. He was now attempting to engage the consumer in a more systematic problem-solving process, an intervention consistent with CBT. Kyle listened attentively to her descriptions of persecution from others, neither agreeing nor disagreeing about their truth. He learned more about her family relationships (she said she felt coddled, and that her father was often harsh and critical), and how she planned to look for work after the probation ended. Kyle encouraged Jacqui to reflect on her current challenges in the context of her goal of returning to work, reminding her that she needed to be careful about how she presented herself to others. Jacqui believed that the social worker sincerely wanted to understand her and had no intentions of using his power for coercive interventions such as referrals for vocational counselling, as others had done at the hospital.

Kyle continued encouraging her ventilation and reflection regarding family and career. He was her trusted confidante, and Jacqui became willing to share personal concerns with him. She was still quite anxious and fearful of others, and had trouble sleeping, so Kyle asked her on occasion if she might want to consider medications. Jacqui was adamant about not taking medications because it would be an acknowledgement that she was mentally ill. Kyle, however, framed the issue of medications as a resource, possibly a short-term one, and one she could control, that might help her deal with the stresses she was experiencing and help her sleep. To his surprise, one month into their relationship Jacqui agreed to accept medications from Dr. Morris—but she wanted it clearly understood that it was only to help her deal with stress caused by others, not because of a mental illness. Kyle agreed, and Dr. Morris prescribed a low-dose antipsychotic medication with antianxiety properties. Interestingly, Jacqui never asked for information about the kind of medication she was taking.

When Jacqui's initial probationary period neared its end, the MHA staff scheduled a hearing. They were hoping for a two-year extension to Jacqui's outpatient probation as a means of demonstrating that this new policy was viable and could be used successfully with other consumers. While neither Kyle nor Dr. Morris was asked to attend the hearing, they were asked to write letters about her participation in the agency's programs and her current mental status. Kyle and the physician agreed that Jacqui was not a threat to herself or to anyone else, so they recommended that her probation be terminated rather than extended. This surprised the MHA, but it was the same decision reached by the judge. Jacqui was now free of legal constraints.

Expanding the Consumer's Perspective

Jacqui and her family were thrilled with this outcome, and grateful to Kyle and Dr. Morris for their roles in the process. Still, Kyle was not sure Jacqui would agree to maintain her involvement with the agency now that it was a voluntary situation. When they had a post-hearing discussion about this, Jacqui said that she wanted to keep meeting with Kyle, so she could "talk to someone about [her] career plans," as she put it. Kyle, of course, supported this decision. It appeared that Jacqui had decided that the kind of assistance she was getting was helpful.

During the following year, which was the duration of Kyle's involvement with Jacqui, he began offering other verbal interventions, including education about job possibilities in the area and a stronger focus on her newly stated personal goals, which included independent living, new social contacts, and a return to church after a long absence. Kyle tentatively provided guidance about these matters, offering opinions, for example, about how she might best make friends and prepare for job interviews. By doing so he was attending to cognitive restructuring, and helping her to consider that some of her negative beliefs about others might be exaggerated. Jacqui was still suspicious of others, but less so, and she became better able to function socially as she visited various Christian churches in her area. Jacqui had been a sporadic churchgoer in the past but felt now that she might benefit from regular fellowship, especially with other Lebanese Americans. She used Kyle as a sounding board when considering any decisions and she continued to take the same dosage of medications, which was helping to control her anxiety and, fortunately, not producing any notable adverse effects.

Still, their work together was conflicted at times. This was most dramatically evident when her mother died suddenly of a heart attack and, in her grief, Jacqui blamed Kyle, saying he had "stressed [her] mother out" too much by "interfering" in their family issues. (Kyle had maintained regular contact with the family, usually supporting Jacqui's progress as her mother and sister complained about her slow movement.) In her grief, Jacqui fired Kyle, who, while upset, dealt with the situation by patiently waiting two weeks before calling her again and asking if they might resume working together. Jacqui agreed, having had several weeks to mourn her mother's death, and never again raised the issue of Kyle's supposed role in the tragedy.

Another time Jacqui asked Kyle to meet with her and her father in their home to support her desire to move out of that apartment, because she was reluctant to confront her volatile father alone. Kyle did so, but as he supported Jacqui's desire for independent living, Michael became angry, shouting profanities at Kyle and ordering him to leave the house. Jacqui appreciated Kyle's advocacy and a few weeks later she invited him back, assuring him that her father had calmed down. Kyle came as invited, and Michael, present as always, made no mention of the incident.

Another source of tension was her sister Rita's ongoing efforts to control Jacqui's behavior. She always believed that

Jacqui was not taking enough medications, and not interacting with the family with sufficient enthusiasm. As always, Kyle empathized with the family's concerns but defended the nature of Jacqui's recovery.

Facilitating New Understandings and Introducing Possibilities for Action

Despite her father and sister's desires to keep Jacqui at home, she did not let go of her desire to become independent. Toward this end she and Kyle continued to utilize a problem-solving format to discuss her goals related to resuming a law practice. Kyle raised the idea of Jacqui's participation in various rehabilitation groups and activities (vocational assessment and counseling, socialization groups, volunteer activities), thinking they might be helpful. She politely declined these options and stated that she understood the legal community and knew best how to gradually reintroduce herself to people who might give her an opportunity to begin practicing again. Kyle supported her efforts but always cautioned her about moving too quickly: Jacqui tended to believe (unrealistically, in his view) that this would be a relatively easy process. Their relationship remained strong. Jacqui considered Kyle to be a confidante and a peer with regard to his understanding of her, his support, and his encouragement of her growth activities. Throughout the entire year, Jacqui never acknowledged that she had a mental disorder, or that any of her thoughts were or had been unrealistic, yet she was not sharing delusional ideas any longer.

Eventually Jacqui found two part-time jobs, different from what she originally had in mind, but jobs in which she felt fulfilled. She was hired by a major commercial tax organization as a processor and worked twenty hours per week in that capacity. The job afforded her a consistent work schedule and allowed her to utilize her taxation expertise. The office was located within walking distance of her home. Next, Jacqui applied for a teaching position at a small local university and became a part-time instructor of taxation. Kyle agreed, at her request, to write her a reference letter toward getting that job.

Jacqui also joined a Christian church where she felt comfortable. After a few months of membership she planned and initiated a monthly discussion group there for area Lebanese professionals, and while this was not successful, surviving for only several months, it helped Jacqui meet more members of that community. Jacqui had never before shown much motivation to develop social relationships outside her family.

Throughout the year, Jacqui never indicated a desire to end her relationship with Kyle, although their frequency of meetings gradually diminished to monthly, by mutual consent. After finding work, her major goal became moving into her own apartment, but she was always ambivalent about this because, despite their conflicts, she was strongly attached to her father. With an opportunity afforded by her new income, she and her father arranged to move into an apartment that was more spacious than the previous one. Jacqui felt that it was "her" apartment, and with the added space she enjoyed greater privacy. As her life settled down, Jacqui took more of an interest in Kyle's life, asking him about his own career goals and giving him advice in that regard. Kyle was careful not to disclose personal information with Jacqui, but appreciated her interest, as they had spent a year talking about a wide range of topics.

Jacqui and Kyle worked together for a total of fifteen months, and their relationship ended when Kyle moved away from the region. He told Jacqui about the move months in advance, and they continued to meet as before. Jacqui was sorry that Kyle was leaving, and she wanted to be transferred to another social worker, to have someone to check in with about how things were going in her life. She also wanted to continue seeing Dr. Morris. Jacqui took Kyle out to lunch for their final session, and he later received complimentary phone calls from both her father and her sister.

Commentary So what characterized this intervention as recovery focused, and how did it differ from traditional social work practice? These questions are answered in the list below, but it should be mentioned first that Kyle saw his work as recovery focused even though Jacqui denied she had a mental illness and would have disagreed that she was recovering from anything. From Kyle's perspective, Jacqui had accepted that she was emotionally vulnerable to high-stress situations, and she had become aware of her need to carefully monitor her emotional well-being, in part with medications, so that she did not have such troubling reactions in the future. Furthermore, Kyle thought that Jacqui might have an awareness that her thoughts became irrational at times, although she never spoke of this. Beyond this, the social worker did the following:

- Made a conscious effort to observe recovery values, the most prominent in this situation being holism, self-direction, empowerment, respect, strengths, responsibility, and hope. (See question #3 at the end of the chapter.)
- Formulated a psychiatric diagnosis for Jacqui but did not base his interventions on it.
- Gave Jacqui the power to determine her own treatment structure.
- Let Jacqui find her own path toward recovery, suggesting no particular goals at the outset.
- Maintained flexible relationship boundaries, while being careful to limit his own self-disclosure. (Some of Kyle's peers worried that he was "too casual" in his interactions with the consumer.)
- Consistently maintained a stance of advocacy with Jacqui, risking conflicts with mental-health-system administrators and her family members in doing so.
- Encouraged her to find normal social supports rather than utilizing those that were part of the formal mental health system.
- At the time of his leaving, the agency let her decide whether she wanted to work with another professional.

In addition to these practices, the social worker also utilized the formal intervention strategies of sustainment, cognitive restructuring, and problem solving.

The following vignette further highlights the relationship-based nature of recovery practice.

The Cyclist

The following intervention took place at a university-affiliated training agency for graduate students in social work and psychology. While modeled after a community mental health center, the agency did not have contract arrangements with any psychiatric hospitals or emergency services facilities, and had only informal linkage agreements with a few psychiatrists for medication evaluations. Supervisors thus discouraged the agency's acceptance of consumers with psychotic disorders. Jason was referred to the agency by his parents, one of whom had a university affiliation. They believed that their twenty-seven-year-old son had a psychotic disorder. The agency director accepted the referral only because one of the supervisors, a licensed clinical social worker, had an interest working with this type of consumer. Adam was an experienced community mental health center practitioner who worked from a recovery philosophy. He was well-known to recovery advocates in the region.

Jason Davis was a single unemployed Caucasian male who lived with his parents. He organized his daily life around training for the Olympic games in the sport of distance cycling. While he was active in the sport locally, Jason had no particular talent and his aspirations to be a world champion were by all accounts, other than his own, unfounded. His parents, in fact, said this "delusion" was a central aspect of their son's odd thinking and behavior. He had been living with them for the past two years, following three postcollege years out of state, and was dependent on them for material and emotional sustenance. When he was not out riding, Jason kept to himself in his room, spending hours each day on the computer researching European racing teams and sending applications to join them. He often complained to his parents of what he called "suspicious activity" in their middle-class neighborhood, and occasionally called the police to report supposed drug-dealing activities going on in the area. These reports were unfounded, and the police had stopped responding to his calls, instead meeting with Jason's parents and asking them to try to curb his behavior.

Jason had a reputation among the neighbors as a harmless kook. His parents asked him to seek counseling for his problems, but Jason refused, stating firmly that there was nothing wrong with him. He acknowledged that he was unhappy, but blamed this on the unsettling activities of his neighbors and the ongoing efforts of his high school friends, none of whom he had seen for years, to send him what he called "negative vibes" to keep him confused. His parents believed strongly that Jason should get help and perhaps take medications, which he had done five years ago during a similar episode. Jason only agreed to cooperate with counselling after his parents offered him $50 per session in spending money to do so.

Engagement

During their first meeting, Adam was struck by the consumer's tangential verbosity, which he called "word salad." (Several of Jason's comments are included in chapter 6.) Adam had difficulty following Jason's train of thought and could not make sense out of his discourses about such things as "mental differences between boys and girls," "the isolative athletic temperament," and his "need for emotional space to work on [his] bicycling repairs." Jason's loose associations continued throughout the hour, and Adam had to repeatedly remind the consumer to stop when their scheduled hour was over. Jason also talked about his concerns related to the malevolent intentions of others, and about his parents' inability to understand his needs. Throughout the interview, the consumer did not make eye contact with Adam, and the nature of his comments were not matched by any changes in his mood. When asked about goals, Jason said that he wanted help in maintaining a life routine that would enable him to be ready for the next Olympics, and for his parents to understand him better. Jason agreed to a series of weekly meetings. (Adam was not aware of the financial arrangement his parents had made with the agency.)

Jason gave Adam permission to talk to his parents, so the social worker called his father for a consult. (Jason perceived such contact as a means for Adam to provide therapy for his father, whom he believed was unbalanced.) Mr. Davis stated that Jason had had a psychotic break as a twenty-one-year-old while living in San Francisco with his brother. He was living there after his college years, where Jason had been doing a lot of drinking and possibly drugs. Mr. Davis suspected that Jason's mental problems had been induced by drug use, and further reported that Jason had been seen as an outpatient by several psychiatrists and treated with a mild dose of antipsychotic medication at that time. While the medications seemed to have calmed Jason then, he never admitted there was anything wrong with him, and he only took his prescriptions for a few months. The young man had lived an isolated existence since then, first on his own but later moving back home when he realized he could not hold a job, and when he ran out of money and was in trouble with local authorities for reporting what he called "neighborhood conspiracies" with some regularity. Jason did not attempt to work after moving back home, but kept to himself and attended to his athletic interests. According to Mr. Davis, Jason began talking about becoming an Olympic athlete a year previously and had organized his life since then around training practices and occasional races in regional events, where he always finished in the middle of the pack. Mrs. Davis was diagnosed with breast cancer around the time of Jason's return. Mr. Davis expressed that he was worried about his wife as well, whose cancer was in remission but still being carefully monitored. He hoped his son could "come to his senses," get a job, and begin spending time with other people.

After the assessment, Adam concluded that Jason's symptom profile was consistent with the criteria for schizoaffective disorder. While Adam did not like to work from a diagnostic perspective, he was required to enter this impression into the consumer's record.

Sustainment and Processing Distress

Because Jason did not acknowledge the presence of a mental disorder, and did not question the practicality of his life activities, Adam was not sure how to proceed with therapy. Jason admitted that he could use some help in formulating his life plans and combating the mental interference he was experiencing from his old high school friends, who were filling him with what he called "negative thoughts." Jason thought he might be able to learn some techniques from the social worker to become less reactive to those events. Adam decided that since Jason was verbal, and they appeared to get along well, he would talk about whatever was on the consumer's mind but encourage him to explore the concerns that created his stress. Perhaps Jason would come to trust the social worker enough to begin considering some of his observations about Jason's broader lifestyle options. Adam believed that, given Jason's history, he might benefit from psychotropic medication, but while he raised the issue as a possibility on a number of occasions as a way for Adam to feel more composed, the consumer always refused, saying that medication was "toxic" to an athlete's system.

Over the course of six weeks, Jason came in for his appointments, usually arriving thirty to forty-five minutes early, and shared concerns about a number of interpersonal problems involving his parents and old friends. Among other things, he talked at length about a young woman whom the consumer had met in a bar, spent one afternoon with, and had not seen again, who he called his "girlfriend." In Jason's words, she had found him to be "weird," "not her type" and "rude." Jason was convinced that she was to be the love of his life, and that she had misunderstood his respectful intentions toward her. He reported seeing the girl frequently (this did not seem rooted in fact), and eventually reported having gone to primary and high school with her, "so it follows we're meant to be together." Jason did not know where the woman lived and had not spoken to her since the first encounter, which he called a "date." Still, he often said that he "needed" to be married and a father by the age of thirty, because many of his relatives had done so, and since he was twenty-seven, "time was running out." Adam responded with empathy but also challenged Jason's reasoning about the nature of his relationship with the girl in an effort to help Jason consider that he might be misperceiving her intentions.

Interestingly, Jason appeared to enjoy his therapy sessions very much, and usually stated at the end, "It really helps to talk things out." Whenever the social worker said anything affirming to Jason, the consumer responded, "Oh, that makes me feel better. Thanks for pointing that out." Jason and Adam were enjoying each other's company, although the consumer's behavior had not changed markedly. In fact, the social worker was asked by the agency director at one point to "talk to him about bothering the waiting room secretary" because Jason, due to his early arrivals, would often initiate "bizarre" conversations with others.

Expanding the Consumer's Perspective

Adam hoped that as Jason developed trust in him, he might eventually consider some of the social worker's alternative perceptions on events surrounding the consumer (such as "Well, Jason, sometimes when people look suspicious they really aren't up to anything criminal, so it's important not to jump to conclusions"). In this way, Adam was addresing Jason's cognitive distortions. One major challenge Adam faced during the first six weeks was that Jason's father called several times to complain about the consumer's angry, insulting behaviors at home toward his parents. Due to his empathizing with Mr. Davis, Adam made a major mistake during their seventh meeting—he not only suggested the idea of medications again (as a way for Jason to control his stress), but also persisted in encouraging the consumer to consider them. Adam had overestimated his level of rapport with the consumer, and Jason became angry. He accused Adam of thinking he was "crazy," and stormed out of the room, saying they were finished.

While shaken by this event, Adam called Jason one week later to invite him to another session. The consumer accepted. When they met again Adam apologized about the prior conversation and admitted he had been wrong for pushing Jason. The consumer accepted the apology, and in fact said it was "no big deal," but Adam wanted Jason to understand that he was free to disagree with the social worker, and that their work should be collaborative. (Adam believed that a part of collaborative practice was admitting to his mistakes and then moving on.) Their sessions resumed as before, with much the same content—training for the Olympics, dealing with life at home, and eventually moving to Europe. At first Jason's plans were all related to cycling—accepting sponsorships from equipment manufacturers, becoming a race director, and possibly working in a bicycle shop. As they discussed the pros and cons of these various possibilities, Jason eventually decided to investigate some local employment, such as working in a repair shop, while he continued to send applications for memberships to European racing teams. It seemed that Jason was becoming open to considering other perspectives on his life plans.

One day, about four months into their work together, Jason surprised Adam by asking if there was a physician he could see about resuming the medications he had taken five years earlier. When Adam asked why, the consumer reported that he had been thinking about it, and decided he could use some help with stress relief, because he and his parents continued to argue frequently. Adam had already been suggesting a variety of relaxation activities for Jason to practice to promote his stress-coping skills. Adam made a referral and helped Jason arrange to see a private practitioner. The psychiatrist, with whom Adam had occasional phone contact from that point, prescribed the same medications Jason had taken years ago, although he first recommended a higher dose than the consumer would accept. Following the introduction of medications, there was no apparent difference in Jason's mental status for several weeks, but gradually Jason became less agitated, even as his unrealistic thoughts persisted.

Facilitating New Understandings and Introducing Possibilities for Action

For the next year Jason and Adam met weekly, and Jason continued to express how helpful the sessions were in terms of being at peace with some of his troubling thoughts. Adam believed that they were productively engaging in a process of person-situation reflection during this time. Jason began bringing notes to each session with a list of topics to cover, checking them off as he went along. There was much repetition in this content, including the themes of relationships with his parents, the lingering influence of his old friends, concerns about getting together with his "girlfriend," and preparing for a career as a professional cyclist. Adam, while recognizing a lack of realism behind many of Jason's goals, provided the consumer with an affirming presence, emphasized his strengths and capabilities, and supported his emerging interest in considering alternative activities if the ones he had in mind did not work out. He encouraged Jason to be patient with making major decisions and to appreciate that everyone's path through life is unique. Adam did not directly confront Jason's delusional ideas because the consumer held to them so strongly, but neither did he affirm their reality.

Adam recognized over time that Jason was strongly attached to his nuclear and extended family, particularly his grandparents. The consumer would often become tearful talk-ing about his aging grandparents and his desires to stay close to them, his desire to reconcile with his parents, and his ongoing concerns about his mother. In fact, it turned out that Jason was a highly emotional young man who had never felt comfortable expressing his feelings. It also became clear that Jason was reluctant to move out of his parents' house, partly because he felt that he needed to be there to support his mother, who con-tinued to undergo cancer treatments, while his father was often out of town on business. Adam tried to help Jason recognize that, while it was admirable that he cared about his family, he also needed to attend to his own goals, and his own individua-tion, and that it might be beneficial for him to talk to his par-ents about his dilemma.

During their second year of work together, Jason experi-enced a fundamental shift in his thinking about the future. He discussed his awareness of the competitive nature of cycling and began wondering if he was young enough to succeed in that arena. He decided he would experiment with other jobs, a deci-sion that Adam strongly supported. At this point, Adam per-ceived that he was helping Jason through the interventions of education and problem solving. Jason began a frustrating search that eventually led to him being hired as a part-time cook in a local delicatessen. Jason enjoyed the work, and his parents were pleased with this development. Still, despite the social worker's encouragement, Jason was unable to establish social relationships there. Adam had been interested to see how Jason's interpersonal skills would evolve, since he was uniformly pleasant and polite. The consumer had considered "making friends" to be a primary goal, but although he was doing well on the job, he kept to himself, describing his coworkers as "too young," "too immature" or "too superficial" to befriend. Adam came to believe that Jason had a natural isolative temperament and would possibly never have many friends.

Jason surprised Adam again six months later by announcing he had decided to pursue a career in cooking, and that he was looking into culinary arts programs. Jason added that he could always continue with his cycling as a hobby and means of exercise, but that he might be better off with a different career. Adam supported this new plan, and learned that Jason's parents did as well, and that his parents had offered him financial support for school. Jason began working on his career goals more closely with his father. Several months later, Jason was accepted into a two-year program in a neighboring state, and became busy making plans to move away. He and Adam agreed to continue meeting when Jason was in town for breaks, and Adam granted the consumer's request to talk by phone from time to time.

During the next year, Jason and Adam met infrequently, but Adam provided a steady supportive presence in the consumer's life. Jason was doing well academically and in his internships, but continued to have little interaction with his classmates or coworkers. In fact, Jason expressed boredom, saying he felt good and kept busy during the week, but was lonely on the weekends. Adam encouraged Jason's social inclinations, and they spent a majority of their time processing this issue and practicing social skills, including role-plays, but this was an area of the consumer's life that remained problematic. Eventually

Jason graduated with high grades and performance reviews and was hired to work at a hotel in San Francisco, where some extended family lived. This represented a major success on the consumer's part, and he was quite pleased. Jason and Adam had a termination session; Jason was, as usual, grateful and complimentary about their time together. Jason then moved away to begin working in San Francisco, and living with an aunt. After he had become settled, Jason called Adam to thank him for his help and to report that he was getting ready to move into his own apartment.

Commentary Jason's intervention unfolded much like the previous example (Jacqui), because the social worker recognized the importance of trust and relationship development with this consumer who did not acknowledge the existence of a mental disorder, although he vaguely recognized a need for assistance in getting his life on track. Given that Jason's case management needs were modest, or not acknowledged, he was appreciative of the social worker's support and was receptive to interventions that can be described as cognitive-behavioral (focused on clarifying thinking process, providing education, and providing problem-solving assistance) and solution focused (helping the client recognize his strengths and develop growth strategies accordingly).

Listed below are highlights regarding the relationship-based nature of Adam's approach with Jason:

- He accepted the consumer as he was, and tried to understand the world from his perspective.
- He used whole person language with Jason and his father rather than clinical jargon.
- He rarely talked specifically about specific symptoms.
- He admitted at a crucial juncture that he had made a mistake, and then apologized for it.
- Rather than close the case when Jason moved away, he made himself available for phone calls and quarterly visits.
- He supported the consumer's career goals and his move even while being concerned that Jason was taking on a great deal of added personal pressure and risked failure.

Jason did seem to see himself at the end of the intervention as recovering from what he called an "emotional breakdown," although he still did not perceive himself as having a mental illness. This was fine with his social worker.

Summary

Schizophrenia (more specifically, schizoaffective disorder) was used in this chapter as an example of a psychotic disorder for which social work recovery practice is appropriate. Among the many ways in which a practitioner might intervene with consumers, the focus of this chapter was on engagement, sustainment and processing distress, expanding the consumer's perspective, facilitating new understandings of challenges, and introducing new possibilities for action. In the next chapter, we will see how recovery practice can be implemented with a different type of consumer, one who experiences depression. The featured examples will include descriptions of a range of holistic interventions that include, but also go beyond, what has been presented in this chapter.

Major Chapter Learning Points

- Schizophrenia is a mental disorder characterized by abnormal patterns of thought and perception. It is considered to be a chronic disorder, one in which symptoms wax and wane over the course of a person's life.
- Recovery from schizophrenia is largely influenced by the person's developing a lifestyle characterized by manageable stress, the presence of supportive others, and structured, productive, activity with moderate levels of stimulation.
- A range of medication and psychosocial interventions have been generated to help persons with schizophrenia achieve symptom relief and improve their social funtioning; they can all assist with the recovery process.
- A major challenge for social workers in recovery practice with persons having schizophrenia is to develop a relationship of trust in spite of the presence of psychotic symptoms.

Questions for Reflection or Discussion

1. Is it possible to engage in recovery-oriented practice with an involuntary consumer who denies that he or she has a mental disorder?

2. To what extent are the social workers' interventions in this chapter focused on relationship development versus other interventions? Does this focus seem appropriate?

3. In the first vignette, to what extent did the social worker, Kyle, observe the values of holism, self-direction, empowerment, respect, strengths, responsibility, and hope?

4. What other approaches or interventions might the social workers have used in each of the two vignettes to help the consumers articulate and work toward a recovery vision?

Chapter 8

Depression

Of all the emotional problems that a person may experience, depression may be the most common. Everyone experiences depression from time to time, although the mood may or may not interfere with one's ability to function. While depression exists on a continuum in terms of severity and persistence, the APA (2000) categorizes two types of depression as representing mental disorders that may benefit from professional intervention: major depression and dysthymic disorder. The purpose of this chapter is to discuss the nature of severe depression and then consider recovery interventions for consumers who experience it.

A major depressive episode is a period of at least two weeks during which a person experiences a depressed mood or loss of interest in nearly all life activities (APA, 2000). Symptoms may be present in the following areas:

- Affect. Sadness, anxiety, anger, irritability, emotional numbness
- Behavior. Agitation, crying, flatness of expression, slowness of physical movement and speech
- Attitudes toward the self. Guilt, shame, low self-esteem, helplessness, pessimism, hopelessness, thoughts of death or suicide
- Cognition. Decreased ability to think and concentrate
- Physiology. Inability to experience pleasure, changes in appetite and sleep patterns, loss of energy, fatigue, decreased sex drive, somatic complaints

Dysthymic disorder represents a personality style featuring symptoms that are similar to but less intense than those of major depression. In dysthymic disorder, the symptoms tend to be chronic but are occasionally remitting.

It is estimated that 16 percent of people in the United States will experience a major depressive disorder in their lifetimes (Kessler, Berglund, et al., 2005), and in a given year 1.5 percent of the adult population will suffer from dysthymic disorder (Kessler, Chiu, Demler, &

Walters, 2005). Many people with depression experience recurrent episodes of the disorder that significantly interfere with their ability to attend to their life responsibilities and interests. These persons are often suitable for recovery-based interventions, because they face ongoing challenges integrating the disorder, however they understand it, into their self-concepts.

A chief limitation of the psychiatric view of depression is the tendency to see it as *only* an internal, biological dysfunction. This can be seen in the widespread acceptance of biological theories of depression and the use of medication as primary treatment. The focus on medication has been criticized by some as a means of providing symptom relief rather than promoting a broader understanding of the phenomenon (Marecek, 2006).

The Experience of Depression

It is important for recovery-oriented practitioners to grasp the human experience of depression. In a landmark qualitative study of thirty persons with lifelong recurrent depression, David Karp (1995) identified four themes in the course of the disorder. This conceptualization is important to recovery practice because it presents a consumer rather than a professional perspective on the experience. The four stages follow:

1. An initial period of inchoate troubling feelings. The person lacks a vocabulary to label his or her troubling experiences. He or she believes "something is not right," but has no clear sense of what is happening, or how to describe it, or that it might represent the beginning of a persistent problem state. The person often assumes that these feelings are related to a transient developmental stage or to external circumstances that will eventually pass. This initial stage of illness identity development may begin at a young age and persist for years. The person tries to cope by diverting his or her attention away from the problem: rather than confront the problem directly, because it is not perceived as a circumscribed problem, the person occupies him- or herself with other activities so as not to be so focused on the troubling mood. Such diversions may include work, hobbies, substance abuse, and other activities, some of which are productive and some of which are potentially harmful.

2. The person concludes, "Something is really wrong with me." For the first time the person perceives his or her negative mood state as related to internal rather than external circumstances. This stage often emerges when a person experiences situational changes with no accompanying change in mood. The person does not yet recognize his or her state as being depression, and is still not sure how to label what is happening, or whether it is an emotional problem. The person attempts to address the problem, alone or with the help of significant others. The person may read, talk to friends, or attempt to use self-reflection to manage the ongoing challenge. Such self-help strategies may be effective in the short run.

3. A crisis brings the person into a world of therapeutic experts. The onset of this stage, unlike the others, is readily identifiable by the person as being related to a crisis of some kind. The person clearly recognizes that he or she needs professional help, although it may be a significant other who convinces the person to seek such help. Many people with chronic depression have high expectations for empathy from professionals. They want someone to listen, help them process their life challenges, and be patient about instituting any formal interventions, such as medication. Sadly, the participants in Karp's study expressed disappointment with most of the professionals they encountered. Over the course of many years, they started and stopped working with many professionals before finding one who had an appropriate orientation toward helping, one that went beyond a medical perspective on the disorder.

4. The person comes to grips with an illness identity. As described above, people who have long-term depression frequently experience a considerable amount of professional intervention, but it does not resolve their depression. The person at some point comes to accept that the depression is chronic, and must evaluate how to live with it, through lifestyle choices as well as, possibly, ongoing professional intervention. The person recognizes that he or she must make sense of it in some way, often through spiritual reflection. The person may not ultimately see him- or herself as having a disorder, but accepts that he or she is a depressed person, which is not the same thing.

To summarize, people with depression are often ambivalent about working with professional practitioners. Karp learned that what people with depression most wanted from a professional was to be listened to and understood. They did not want the professional to rush into any type of formal intervention. This perspective supports the recovery philosophy of practice, a collaborative encounter in which consumers are helped to organize a satisfactory life in spite of the presence of an ongoing mental, emotional, and behavioral challenge.

Before describing recovery practice strategies that may be utilized with persons who are depressed, some research-based findings related to the nature of depression and its course are presented.

Risk and Resilience Influences for Depression

Biological Influences   The fact that major depression tends to run in families partially supports the notion of genetic transmission for some persons. The extent of variance that heritability explains for major depression ranges from 31 to 42 percent (Sullivan, Neale, & Kendler, 2000). Many types of depression are thought to be associated with deficiencies of certain neurotransmitters in the limbic area of the brain, which controls emotions. Although no genes have been found to have more than small effects, studies have centered on the serotonin transporter gene (Kumsta et al., 2010) and its interaction with stressful life events (Caspi et al., 2003).

Psychological Influences   At the psychological level, depression is often related to distorted and rigid beliefs and thoughts that are self-critical. These typically involve the cognitive triad of depression: thoughts about the self as worthless, the world as unfair, and the future as hopeless (Beck, Rush, Shaw, & Emery, 1979). Coping style is another psychological variable associated with the onset of depression. Coping methods that are more active in nature, such as problem solving, have the potential to ward off depression. Avoidant coping styles, such as evading situations and indulging in ruminative thinking, such as focusing on symptoms in a passive way, present risk (Nolen-Hoeksema, 2002).

Social Influences   Family factors can influence the development of depression in youth. The absence of parental warmth and availability has been particularly associated with depression (McLeod, Weisz, & Wood,

2007). The association of parental depression with increased rates of depression in children may be accounted for by genetics, biological impairment transmitted from mother to developing fetus, dysfunctional parenting, modeling, and parental marital problems (Goodman, 2007).

A number of studies have indicated a significant relationship between depression and childhood physical and sexual abuse (Penza, Heim, & Nemeroff, 2006). Of all types of maltreatment, sexual abuse poses the greatest risk for depression (Fergusson, Boden, & Horwood, 2008). Adults who reported being maltreated as children appear to have an elevated inflammatory response to stress compared to adults who lacked mistreatment in their histories, thus childhood maltreatment may create a biological vulnerability to depression (Carpenter et al., 2010). Other family relationships may influence the development of depression. For adults, those who were divorced or separated were more likely to experience major depression in the past year (13.1 percent) than were people in other relationship status categories (SAMHSA, 2009). Conversely, sibling affection and support may play a protective role (Padilla-Walker, Harper, & Jensen, 2010).

In general, social support may mitigate harsh family circumstances and the stressful life events that people with depression are prone to experience (Kraaij, Arensman, & Spinhoven, 2002). Friends can provide support and enable people to self-disclose in a safe setting. Having supportive peers is associated with less depression in adolescence (Gutman & Sameroff, 2004), whereas higher frequencies of bullying (physical, verbal, or relational) have a linear relationship to levels of depression (Wang, Iannotti, Luk, & Nansel, 2010). For girls, relational victimization, when paired with genetic vulnerability, is predictive of depression (Benjet, Thompson, & Gotib, 2010). In terms of the wider social environment, one systematic review found that socioeconomic status holds a negative association with depression for youth aged ten to fifteen years (Lemstra et al., 2008).

What follows is an overview of interventions for depression.

Standard Interventions

Almost two-thirds of adults who experienced major depression received treatment in the past year (SAMHSA, 2009). Many such persons seek help from the general health system, however, and as a result only about

19 percent of this group receive appropriate care, defined as services that are consistent with empirically validated treatment guidelines (Young, Klap, Sherbourne, & Wells, 2001). There is more reliance on medication than on psychotherapy in the general health system (Olfson & Marcus, 2009). If the practitioner concludes that the risk of suicidal behavior is considerable, he or she should consider inpatient treatment. Outpatient intervention is indicated if the consumer is free of psychosis, not abusing substances, and maintaining control over suicidal thoughts. After suicide risk has been assessed, interventions for persons with depression may include psychotherapy and medication. A recent trend has been for physicians to prescribe the latter more frequently than the former (Olfson & Marcus, 2009). Medication is considered to act on the biological mechanisms of depression, but it must be recognized that psychotherapy may also produce positive biological changes.

Psychotherapy

The benefits of psychotherapy are that many consumers prefer it to medication (Karasu, Gelenberg, Merriam, & Wang, 2002). Psychotherapy is particularly indicated when the person's life is characterized by psychosocial stress, difficulty coping, and interpersonal problems. Psychotherapies with considerable research support include CBT and interpersonal therapy (IPT). CBT involves behavioral models that focus on the development of coping skills, especially in the domains of social skills and daily activities, so that the person receives more reinforcement from his or her environment. Cognitive models include assessing and changing the distorted thinking that people with depression may exhibit. Although typically delivered as a package of interventions, some of these techniques have been used as stand-alone treatment. Examples are behavioral activation, which centers on activity scheduling and increasing pleasant activities; and problem solving, which focuses on behaviorally defining specific problems, brainstorming ideas to solve them, and deciding on solutions. IPT is an intervention that focuses on how current interpersonal relationships have contributed to the person's depression. The social worker's goal is to help the consumer repair these interpersonal conflicts (Weissman, Markowitz, & Klerman, 2000). Intervention focuses on the consumer's role transitions, grief processes, interpersonal disputes, or deficits.

Various psychotherapies for depression in adults were compared in a meta-analysis (Cuijpers, van Straten, Andersson, & van Oppen, 2008). These included IPT; psychodynamic therapy; nondirective supportive treatment, such as offering empathy and helping people to ventilate their experiences and emotions; CBT; behavioral activation treatment; and problem-solving therapy. None of the treatments was appreciably more efficacious than the others, except for IPT, which was slightly superior to the others.

Medication

The use of antidepressants has increased drastically in recent years, from 5.8 percent in 1996 to 10.1 percent of depressed persons in the United States in 2005 (Olfson & Marcus, 2009), and the use of antipsychotics for depression has increased for both adults and children (Olfson, Blanco, Liu, Moreno, & Laje, 2006). Social workers should be prepared to educate consumers and their families about the benefits and limitations of medication. Close monitoring produces greater treatment adherence and more opportunities for education.

What follows are two illustrations of recovery practice with persons who experience recurrent episodes of major depression. One difference from the vignettes presented in the last chapter is that these consumers found strength after accepting that they had mental illnesses, and were able to come to terms with that fact in productive ways.

The Track Coach

Steve, a social worker, first met Barbara Jamison on the acute care unit of the state psychiatric hospital. Barbara was a sixty-five-year-old married Caucasian woman who had been admitted for a major depressive episode, her fourth admission in the past thirty years. When Steve approached Barbara, she was slumped onto the surface of a table in the cafeteria, not moving, and was unable to make eye contact with him. He introduced himself as the social worker from the community mental health center. Barbara looked up, seeming lost. "Oh, no, you're here, too. What did you do to deserve this?" Steve asked for clarification. "We're all trapped on this submarine. Don't you see, we're lost at the bottom of the ocean. No one will ever find us here. We're doomed."

After a few minutes of trying to talk with Barbara, who was barely able to respond to his questions, Steve returned to the hospital social worker's office, who had called him about working with the consumer after discharge. "Don't be fooled by her," she said. "This is one dynamic woman. She raised four kids and ran a track club in her neighborhood for twenty years. She was the lady in charge, organizing the league, hiring the coaches, and scheduling the meets. Dozens of those kids went on to run track in college. She's got a lot going for her." Steve was surprised to hear this, because Barbara's presentation suggested nothing of the sort. The hospital social worker estimated that the consumer would be in the hospital for several weeks, because she was being started on a regimen of medications before being discharged to her husband, with whom she shared a modest home.

Engagement

Barbara's diagnosis was that of major depressive disorder, recurrent, with psychotic features and full interepisode recovery. During the next two weeks, her mental status gradually improved. She continued to be delusional, flat, and disengaged, but she gained energy and was at least going through the motions of the hospital milieu. Steve visited her twice for short but more substantive conversations, and decided to take this time to get to know her husband. He invited Mr. Jamison to his office for a consultation. Mr. Jamison arrived with one of their four children, a thirty-year-old single daughter named Clara.

Mr. Jamison became tearful as he described his wife's history of depression. "Yes, she gets depressed a lot, not all the time but every few months, and it doesn't help that she wants to lie in bed or sit in a chair all day. I try my hardest to get her motivated. I encourage her to get up, and get out, and think about the kids and me. She won't listen. Usually she snaps out of her low moods after a few weeks, but there have been a few times when I had to call the doctors and get her into the hospital, since she absolutely wouldn't get out of bed or respond to me at all, and she'd talk about wanting to die." Barbara had not, however, made any actively suicidal gestures. His daughter agreed with Mr. Jamison's assessment. "I'll admit to going into her room once in a while and pulling her out of bed, and dragging her out the door, and locking her out of the room, so she has no choice but to come downstairs and be with us. Some people might say we're hard on her, but she needs tough love, and it works, because she's not a strong person."

Steve concluded by the end of the hour that the Jamison family had little understanding of the nature of depression, and that they were interpreting her withdrawal as personal weakness, something that needed to be dealt with by confrontation—and possibly abuse. Barbara was, by their account, a good mother and an attentive wife much of the time, but when depressed, she became isolative, which the family perceived as willful rejection.

The Jamisons had both grown up in a small rural town and had little knowledge of mental illness. Following each of her previous three hospitalizations Barbara had been prescribed antidepressant medication but Mr. Jamison was reluctant to approve of his wife's taking it, thinking it was what he called a "Band-Aid strategy" that did nothing to help her learn how to be a stronger person. For this reason, Barbara usually went off her medications a few months after starting them, and she never attended more than one or two counseling appointments. According to Clara, all four of the children resented what they called her "spells," and had better relationships with their father than with their mother.

Steve believed that the family was well-meaning, but he had concerns about their possible physical abuse of Barbara. For the moment, he decided to focus on Barbara's preparations for discharge. The consumer had brightened up considerably by the end of her second week at the hospital, no longer experiencing delusions, and Steve had time to get to know her. Barbara was different from the person she had been when he had met her. She appeared to be a sociable, caring person, with a kindly grandmother persona. Nevertheless, she had very low self-esteem. "I'm a failure, I know that. I've been a bad wife and a bad mother. I just haven't been there for my family when they needed me. I feel terrible about all that, and I'll have to live with it." Barbara was a religious person who seemed to derive great comfort from her Christian church affiliation. "I pray to God that I can become a better person, a stronger person. I pray that he'll forgive me for my sins. I know he loves me even though I've been a disappointment in so many ways." Steve concluded that Barbara had internalized her family's perception of her as being weak rather than ill. He suggested that her moods might not always be under her control, that she might have a condition that brings on her low moods without personal strength being a factor. Barbara admitted she had heard this before. "That's what they tell me when I come to the hospital, and when I see a doctor for medication he'll sometimes say that, too. I don't really agree. Isn't it everyone's job to try to make me feel better when I'm here?"

Sustainment and Processing Distress

Following Barbara's discharge, she and Steve began a five-year working relationship with the following goals that she articulated:

- Finding purpose in her life with the children gone from the house
- Defining herself in more positive terms
- Accepting her mood problems as chronic but not a reflection of weak character
- Forgiving herself for past regrets
- Forgiving those who she came to believe as having mistreated her
- Engaging in service activities through which she could serve God

Steve's first task was to build a treatment relationship with the consumer and her husband that was not solely focused on medication. He took time to get to know them both through the weekly sessions they attended for three months. Steve educated them about moods and their nature, including their biology, to help them understand that Barbara's depressions were at times out of her control. Steve wanted her husband to understand that during those times, Barbara would not respond to coercion, and in fact that might make her feel worse. Fortunately for Steve, he liked both the Jamisons, and, after some initial misgivings about Mr. Jamison's harsh attitudes, came to believe that he was a man who cared about his wife and believed he was doing the right thing. Mr. Jamison felt incapable of caring for himself and the family on his own, so he became frightened when his wife withdrew. Steve continued educating the couple about the biological basis of Barbara's depressions. At the same time, he affirmed each of their past efforts to deal with the mood changes because he did not want them to feel guilty or ashamed about what had transpired. Steve hoped that his information about depression would help Barbara overcome the stigma she experienced, and become more self-accepting. In essence, Steve helped Barbara to come to terms with an illness identity, accepting that she needed to be aware of her emotional swings but not to assume that they were evidence of weak character. Mr. Jamison had a harder time accepting this disease model of depression, which in this instance would be helpful to the family's relationships, although he tried to understand.

Expanding the Consumer's Perspective

After the initial three months, Steve worked mostly alone with Barbara, although her husband occasionally attended their meetings. Barbara came to accept her depression as biological in origin, but wanted to learn how to control her moods more effectively. She also wanted to develop a lifestyle that was more focused on extra-family community involvement. Her husband, however, despite his good intentions, still could not accept that her moods were related to a disorder. Furthermore, as a retired man with few friends and interests of his own, he wanted Barbara to continue functioning as a stay-at-home wife. He discouraged her interests in other activities, and he was suspicious of the ways in which her deepening spirituality, rooted in their shared Christian faith, was pulling her in a direction of outside service. Barbara recalled her years of running the track club and believed she was capable of making additional contributions to her community. In short, Barbara was learning that her mood problem was not a character flaw, and she was in a process of redefining herself as a good person, rather than a bad wife and mother, who needed to adjust to a disability.

It was during this time that Steve formally introduced the idea of recovery to the Jamisons. As a part of their education, he emphasized that Barbara's depression seemed to be a chronic characteristic, but not all of who she was. He suggested that Barbara could perhaps most fully recover from her mood challenges by taking care of her tendencies toward depession even as she moved beyond them, rather than setting out to eradicate the recurrent condition, which is what her husband wanted her to do. Steve explained that there was a growing recovery community in their city that provided certain resources, including peer support groups, that Barbara might choose to access. Barbara listened with interest, but did not seem ready to act on this information yet.

Facilitating New Understandings and Introducing Possibilities for Action

During their individual sessions, Barbara described to Steve how she and her husband, despite their ongoing commitment to one another, had always been at odds: "He likes being the head of the household, making all the decisions. This is how it always was in our family, and when our kids were growing up I pretty much obeyed him. He's a good man, and always cared about the children, but I never felt that he really cared about me. There were times when he slapped me. I never thought it was wrong when it was happening, because I thought I deserved it, but now I don't think so. When my depression acted up, I would sit around the house like a vegetable, and he used to yell at me to 'shape up,' and slap me until I got out of my chair and started doing housework. He encouraged my kids to treat me the same way. You know my daughter, who you met? She used to yell at me and slug me in the gut, and tell me what a terrible mother I was. I can remember both of them standing over me and yelling until I tried harder to move. That was my life for many years, and I bought into it."

Steve brought up the fact that she had been effective managing the track club, and suggested that since her children turned out well she must have been a pretty good mother, too. Barbara replied, "I was involved with my kids and their friends. I admit that I always wanted to participate in their lives without my husband, because he never seemed to approve of me. That's one reason I got the track club going. It was all mine, and it got me out of the house." Steve asked what kind of future life Barbara envisioned with her family, and she was candid in her response. "I get along well enough with my husband that I don't want to leave him. I'm not sure I could take care of myself anyway. I guess you could say he's more like a roommate than anything else. I want to develop my own interests. I want to use my counseling here to make some decisions about that."

It is important to emphasize here the strength of Steve and Barbara's relationship. Barbara saw the social worker as a "good son" who was pleasant, affirming, and willing to make Barbara's wishes a priority, a process that she was clearly not accustomed to. Steve was impressed with her willingness to self-disclose and trust him to keep this information confidential. They spent the first several months of their individual meetings, scheduled every two weeks, processing her family history and her emerging new identity, and monitoring her medications with an agency physician. Steve was more self-disclosive with Barbara than with most of his other consumers, primarily because he interpreted her inquiries into his life as based on appropriate curiosity. He answered her questions with varying degrees of detail about his family life, growing-up years, and interests. He was careful about what he shared with Barbara, but was comfortable telling her, for example, about his own children and their schooling. These were topics Barbara liked to share about her own children as well, and these exchanges helped to solidify their relationship.

As the months went on, and Barbara stabilized, Steve expressed a desire to help the consumer focus more intently on her personal goals. Barbara emphasized first that she had always been a religious person but wanted to become more active with her Christian faith, offering assistance to her church. Steve helped her to think about ways she might accomplish this and encouraged her to meet with the parish pastor to explore the possibilities. Barbara did so and decided that she would like to become a visitor to the shut-in older adults, providing them with companionship and delivering items prepared by a church council. She also agreed to be a driver on Sundays, taking people without transportation to church services and classes. Behaving like her former energetic self, Barbara quickly became a well-known figure around the parish, and with her excellent social skills and good humor was effective in those roles. She said, "I know God will forgive me for my years of sloth [still reluctant to assume that she had a mental illness] whether I do these things or not, but I think it's important to contribute to the community." She added, "I don't think my family will ever accept me as a good person, but maybe I am in some ways."

This last statement reflected a dilemma that Barbara frequently expressed: how to interact well with her family after so many years of conflict. She had accepted living with her husband as a companion, but she was less sure about her relationships with the children. They were all grown and had moved away, and while they kept in touch with their parents, they still seemed (in Barbara's eyes) to favor their father and to resent her. She decided to limit her efforts to reconnect with the children to weekend phone calls. She hoped this practice might change their attitudes about her, but she did not want to do anything extreme to try to repair those relationships. Steve affirmed this as a reasonable strategy.

Barbara also began asking about the recovery resources that Steve had mentioned from time to time. He reviewed various activities available in their community, and Barbara decided to join a WRAP group. Through this experience she was able to further normalize her experience of depression and infuse activities into her daily routine that would secure her ability to stabilize and transcend her mood. Barbara also became interested in the county MHA and thought that she might like to volunteer there in the future.

Barbara's recovery unfolded steadily over a period of several years. Steve continued to be Barbara's sounding board and a good listener as she continued to seek his advice about her plans, although he found her judgment to be generally good. Barbara was feeling increasingly confident and happy with herself, but then she learned her husband had cancer and would probably only live for six more months.

The word "crisis" can be translated as "a dangerous opportunity," and this is how Barbara viewed her husband's impending death. She maintained a surprisingly positive attitude about helping him through his final months, attributing her religious faith as being her major support, and set out to plan for a life alone after his death. For five months she took care of him at home and arranged for relatives and friends to visit. She and her husband did not have any final words with each other; Barbara had accepted long ago that theirs was not an emotionally intimate relationship. On the day he passed away, his memorial plans were in place. Barbara helped her children grieve and seemed to reconnect with them more strongly during this time.

Barbara continued living in their small house so that she could maintain a home base for the children and ties to the community. By now, Barbara had no fears of living alone; she had learned that she had been a strong woman all along and was quite capable of taking care of herself. She resumed her church activities almost immediately after her husband's death. Barbara continued to meet with Steve every two weeks to process her feelings during these months and she soon expanded her range of social activities.

Four months after her husband's death, Barbara asked Steve for the name of a contact person at the county MHA. She wanted to volunteer her time as a facilitator of a women's depression support group. Steve had told Barbara about such support groups for her to consider as a consumer, but Barbara had not felt she had the time. Now that she was alone, Steve reminded her of this possibility, and Barbara decided she would like to become a facilitator. Steve took her downtown to the MHA offices for an interview with a program director he knew. Barbara was invited to become a volunteer, but not a group facilitator. The program director suggested that she provide volunteer services in the office and join the women's depression support group as a consumer. If Barbara continued to enjoy the group and showed leadership potential in the eyes of the staff, she might be considered for a coleadership role when an opening became available. This was agreeable to Barbara, and signaled the beginning of her long association with that advocacy association.

Barbara continued to use antidepressant medications successfully, and for the next two years did not experience a significant depressed mood. She maintained contact with Steve on a monthly basis, although by this time Barbara primarily used the time to fill in the social worker on her life activities. Steve left the agency after they had worked together for five years; before he left, he transferred the consumer to another social worker, believing that she would function well with minimal support. Barbara acknowledged the ending of the relationship by bringing in a plate of baked goods for Steve to share with his family. Her final advice to him: "Always be good to your mother."

Commentary   Barbara provides a good example of a person whose ability to deal with depression was initially hampered by the fact that she believed herself to be psychologically weak, rather than experiencing a mental disorder. She had never lived among people who understood that her low moods were treatable with counseling and medications. Once she realized that hers was a condition that was not only treatable, but also one around which she might organize a long-range recovery plan, she rallied quickly and was able to apply her considerable strengths and talents toward recovery. Ultimately she became an advocate for persons like herself who might be feeling oppressed by their condition.

Another interesting facet of this intervention is that Steve was rather open with his consumer about his own personal life, although he never shared any of his personal problems. He viewed their work together as a partnership, and as part of his ongoing assessment came to understand that his self-disclosures would help Barbara see that she was in the presence of a collaborator who treated her as a normal, regular person. Some consumers are affected negatively learning about the practitioner's personal life, seeing him or her as being in need of care, or thinking that the practitioner might not be trusted with the consumers' own personal information. This was not true of Barbara.

In summary, Steve's work can be seen as recovery focused in that he

- Increased Barbara's self-esteem and sense of empowerment by teaching her that depression was largely a biological rather than psychological condition, which she had never considered;
- Demonstrated that one could have a mental illness but pursue normal activities;
- Provided education to Barbara's husband in an effort to increase his own understanding of his wife's challenges;
- Maintained a strengths perspective in organizing his case management activities, as he connected the client with the recovery community, her church, and the MHA;
- Engaged in considerable self-disclosure in a conscious effort to help Barbara see them as partners in her recovery; and
- Introduced Barbara to the recovery community as a means of expanding her sense of purpose.

The Photographer

Mike Hollmann was a thirty-year-old German American male who lived with three roommates, none of whom was a close friend. Beginning in adolescence, he had experienced chronic major depression, which he readily admitted required continuous monitoring. Unlike Barbara, Mike became self-destructive when depressed and had attempted suicide a half dozen times. He did not experience psychotic symptoms but withdrew to his bed, lonely and overwhelmed with hopelessness. Because he had no close friends and was estranged from his parents and older sister, who believed him to be a failure as a son and family member, Mike had few supports. Mike had worked at a series of unskilled jobs after graduating from high school, but he usually lost them after periods of missed work related to his depression. Feeling ashamed, Mike would never let his employers know about his disability, and simply stopped going to work. To make matters worse for his confidence, Mike was homosexual in a family and community that still had negative attitudes about that behavior.

Mike was referred to the mental health center following his most recent suicide attempt, after which he had been hospitalized for three weeks. He had seriously cut his wrists and could have died, had a roommate not found him in time. Mike had begun to recover from his low mood while at the hospital with an adjustment in his medications, but he still felt a great deal of shame about upsetting his family and employers (who had not known about his history). Upon entering his treatment program, Mike presented as a sad, broken young man with no apparent future, and who was not altogether sure that he wanted to continue the fight.

He was also in Stage 3 of Karp's illness identity development, searching for the right professional. He had seen many therapists over the years, but had not developed an attachment to any of them. Mike did not think anyone understood him.

Engagement

Mike's social worker was Brian, a same-age African American male. In their first few conversations, Brian sensed that the consumer was always trying to prove himself to be a worthwhile young man, to other persons but also to himself. Mike always summarized his weekly activities rather defensively and intellectually, saying he was taking care of himself, eating well, taking his medications, trying to get out of the apartment regularly, thinking about looking for jobs, and fighting off tendencies toward low moods. Yet Brian could not sense any real motivation in Mike's comments. Brian concluded that Mike had an idea of how he "should" present himselr to be a "good consumer," and the social worker discouraged this attitude. He encouraged Mike to slow down in their conversations, and not press too hard to get back into a busy routine, since it was the pressure of fulfilling structured activities that had contributed to Mike's depressions. Brian affirmed that Mike was doing his best, that he didn't want to struggle so much with self-care, but the social worker added that Mike deserved to take his time, given that he was recovering from a suicidal depression. Brian suggested that Mike give patient thought to what he wanted to do next with his life. Mike agreed that the people around him, especially his family, were always encouraging him to "hurry up" with developing a career path, since they believed it should not be so difficult. Brian supported the consumer's view of the depression as biological, and suggested that Mike think carefully about his strengths and personal goals before rushing into any major new life activities. After their first several visits, Mike seemed to relax, talk more honestly about his challenges, and admit that he felt terrible about himself and relied on other people to tell him what was best. Brian replied that only Mike knew what was best for him, and that the social worker's role would be to help Mike thoughtfully plan for whatever he decided to do.

Expanding the Consumer's Perspective

It took Mike months to trust the commitment of his social worker, but he articulated early on that he wanted to find a job, any job, before thinking about interpersonal goals. His major interpersonal goal did not involve making friends, because Mike did not care about being sociable; rather, he wanted to reconcile the conflicted relationships within his family. Mike accepted Brian's suggestion of a referral to a local vocational assessment program, but he talked with more enthusiasm about his emerging interests in photography and video recording. Brian helped Mike with his immediate job needs but suspected that some type of work in photography represented his real vision.

Mike explained that since adolescence he had been a fan of popular television shows and took a great interest in how they were produced. He taught himself about taping and editing techniques, as well as photography, and invested what money he had into related equipment. This was initially a hobby, but during the months after his hospital discharge Mike took the initiative to undertake a correspondence with the writers and producers of several of his favorite television shows. Before long he was having regular mail contact with the producers of one of television's highest-rated shows, and he loved telling Brian about his latest conversations with them. In the meantime, Brian was enjoying a comfortable relationship with Mike and was helping the doctor monitor his medications. Brian never underestimated the strength of Mike's depressive episodes, but during their initial six months together it was clear that his new hobbies were energizing the consumer. All of Mike's time was now going into either his vocational rehabilitation program or his hobbies. He spent no time with his family and had only superficially cordial relationships with his roommates, and this seemed to suit him.

Mike finished his vocational training program and was offered a part-time job stocking shelves in a supermarket. He accepted the job with gratitude, and functioned well there, but he derived no satisfaction from the work. He admitted that it was boring, but said he needed to live, and besides, in his experience not many people seemed to like their jobs. Mike kept his distance from the other store employees but his tendencies toward depression were known to his employers; Brian encouraged him to make this disclosure, and he was not happy about doing so. Brian was concerned that despite Mike's return to work he was in the kind of dead-end job that might contribute to his depressed moods.

Facilitating New Understandings and Introducing Possibilities for Action

Brian noticed a paradox in his recovery practice with Mike. The consumer wanted to move in the direction of a vocation that touched on his interests while being rehabilitated as a grocery store clerk. He wondered if Mike wanted to pursue his major interests more seriously, now that he had a paying job to support himself. Brian was aware that the local high schools all had audiovisual departments and he wondered if Mike would be interested in approaching the schools as a place to get volunteer experience. Mike was ambivalent about this idea; although it appealed to him, he realized he would need to substantively interact with other people and present himself for a formal interview. Both situations involved skills he did not possess. This was a turning point in Mike's recovery, and what led him to now prioritize the goal of developing social skills: his confidence was growing.

Brian instituted twelve weeks of IPT with Mike, a structured intervention for persons with depression that focuses on resolving interpersonal issues that contribute to the mood problem (Weissman et al., 2000). Brian suggested that the skills Mike practiced in this intervention might also transfer well to future efforts he might make to reconcile with his family. Mike was not ready to take up his family issues, but agreed to engage in IPT.

IPT assumes that mood disorders are medical illnesses but that they are manifested in the consumer's quality of social functioning. There is a relationship between the onset of mood episodes and the nature of a consumer's interpersonal relationships, so the goal of IPT is to enhance the consumer's mastery of interpersonal situations. One of the four foci of the intervention is interpersonal deficits—relationships that are impoverished in terms of number and quality. Brian and Mike worked on reducing his social isolation and encouraging his formulation of new relationships by relating Mike's symptoms in part to a lack of social fulfillment, reviewing the positive and negative aspects of past relationships, and practicing skills to develop new relationships.

Following the IPT intervention, Mike tentatively decided to look for work related to his new interests. Mike was a determined job seeker when he wanted to be, and even though the social worker used his own contacts to check on openings, it was the consumer who learned that one local high school was opening a new audiovisual arts department. Mike contacted the school and arranged for an interview as a possible volunteer. His enthusiasm and skills were so striking to the faculty that he was accepted as a volunteer. He continued to work at the grocery store but also devoted twenty hours per week to the high school, making his weekdays quite busy. This went on for six months, during which time his counseling with Brian continued its focus on social skill development, healthy lifestyle development, and medication monitoring.

A job opening became available at the high school for an activities assistant, whose broad roles would include janitoring, helping to manage the varsity sports teams, and assisting in the production of school plays and internal television productions. Mike talked with Brian about how he might best present himself in an interview for the job, and whether he should inform the staff of his psychiatric history. Brian did not overtly recommend that Mike disclose his history, but he urged the consumer to consider doing so if he believed the staff would be supportive. "Well, they like me, because I always give them more than they require, and I do a good job, so maybe they'd be okay with my condition. If I have problems they might help me rather than fire me." Mike disclosed the history of his depression, and was offered the job, although his supervisor gave him a stern warning: "I don't want to know the details of your personal life, but I do ask that if you begin to get so depressed that it affects your job performance, you let me know." Mike was pleased and quit the grocery store job. From that time forward, Brian worked with Mike on determining when, to whom, and how much he wanted to disclose about his mental health and recovery history. Mike was quite sensitive to his limitation, and carried much stigma about his condition, but he began making some proactive decisions about whom he could confide in besides his social worker and doctor.

Sustainment and Processing Distress

At this time, Mike also decided that he wanted to reconcile with his family. He was anxious about this step because he had been out of touch with his father, sister, and mother for several years, and their last encounters had been negative. The Hollmanns were a culturally nonexpressive family, tending to hold high standards of self-sufficiency, self-control, and productivity. They did not understand that there might be a biological reason for Mike's moodiness and withdrawal. Mike tended to shout when upset, and they believed he was ungrateful for their affections. Furthermore, Mike's father did not accept that he was homosexual. Mike decided to begin with his sister, with whom his relationship was less conflicted. He practiced the social skills he had learned through IPT with Brian through role-playing, and he soon contacted his sister to arrange for a lunch meeting. Mike felt strongly that they should meet in a nice restaurant because he wanted to convey to his sister the seriousness of his willingness to reconcile.

During his first session after that meeting, Mike was upset because the dinner had not gone well. He believed he had tried hard to be thoughtful and calm with his sister as he described his challenges in dealing with depression and also his caring for his family. His sister had been empathic, but not forgiving. She told her brother that from now on he should be a loyal brother and son to make up for the "lost years" of his alienation from them all. Mike tried to accept her lack of awareness of the biology of mental illness, but it was hard for him to remain congenial when she began making demands that he felt were missing the point of what he had been through. At the end of the dinner, they agreed to stay in touch, but she warned Mike not to come over to her house until he had first spoken to their father. She did not want to risk alienating her father by being seen as taking sides against him.

Brian believed that this meeting, while not a complete success, represented a good starting point for resuming his family relationships. It was hard for Mike to accept this idea, however, since he felt he had come a long way and wanted to be understood in ways that were, as he put it, "rational." In time, Mike accepted that he might only make slow progress with his sister, and, feeling more encouraged by Brian's perspective, decided to call his father. Unfortunately, Mike's father refused to accept the call. Mike was devastated and became more depressed. He missed several meetings with the social worker who, because of his concerns about the consumer's situation, aggressively followed up these missed visits with phone calls. When his first few calls were not returned, Brian stopped by Mike's apartment, but either no one was home or he did not answer. Brian continued to call daily and stopped by the apartment every few days.

Mike's withdrawal lasted for two weeks, and he missed several days of work at the school without notifying his supervisor. Mike might have been fired except that his supervisor decided to give the situation some time. Mike eventually called Brian and resumed their meetings. Fortunately he had been taking his medication. Next, Mike went to the high school to face his employer, who was willing to have him come back, but not without an angry warning. "You agreed to let me know if your depression was getting out of control, and you didn't do that. I expect more from you in the future, Mike. You have to take care of your responsibilities if you want to keep any job. We want you here, because you're good, but we need to be able to rely on you. Can we do that? I'm afraid you're going to have to prove it to me." In processing this conversation with the social worker, Mike resolved not to let himself cut off contact with all people again should he become depressed, because he loved his work so much. Of course, hopelessness is a symptom of depression, and at those times a person may not be able to reach out, but the social worker tried to help Mike emphasize the point with a commitment to treatment contract. This is a handwritten form that a consumer fills out and signs, as does the social worker, in which he or she agrees to persist with the intervention agreement even when feeling unmotivated (Joiner, Orden, Witte, & Rudd, 2009). The agreement lays out in writing the steps a consumer agrees to take to ensure that he or she does not discontinue the intervention process at a time when the depression is most acute.

After this crisis episode passed, Mike continued with his pattern of seeing the social worker every two weeks for support, seeing the physician once per month for medication monitoring, and working at the high school. Mike received particularly strong positive feedback when he was able to form a linkage between the producers of a television show with the school's audiovisual department. The producers actually made the high school one of their community service projects, and the association garnered some local press coverage. Mike never did reconcile with his parents, and he talked to his sister only rarely.

Over the months he found different roommates but still did not develop close friends. He was pleased with his relatively stable mental status and the work he was doing. While lonely, he had learned to live on his own and tolerated the situation well. Three years after the beginning of his therapy, he was recovering nicely.

Interestingly, Mike never discussed his homosexuality in any detail with the social worker. Brian raised the issue several times, but Mike politely declined to discuss it. "I can handle that on my own," he said. Brian suspected that Mike carried guilt about his sexual orientation, due to the community culture he had been raised in, and thought it might do his consumer some good to process the issue in their work together. But while Mike was open to discussing most everything else, he did not want to discuss this. Perhaps it is an issue he would face in the future.

Commentary   Mike experienced a major change in life direction during his recovery intervention. The severity of his depressive episodes had rendered him unable to manage any kind of career-related work, and he instead got by with unskilled jobs that provided him with sustenance but nothing in the way of fulfillment. Because he had been estranged from his family and had few friends, he had no compelling purpose for living until the social worker encouraged him to actively pursue his dormant interests and develop them into career opportunities. His social skills improved somewhat with the formal intervention of IPT, and his motivation to connect with his family grew, although he was not successful in reaching his goals in those areas. Still, he had accepted the biological basis of his mood fluctuations and learned that his strengths were such that others could have confidence in him as a contributing member of society. He was less isolative in that he learned to confide in a supervisor and enjoy the students with whom he worked.

Additionally, Brian's work with Mike was recovery focused as he helped the consumer

- Overcome his tendency to present himself to professionals in ways he thought they expected,
- Articulate a true rather than a "false" vision,

- Experience less self-stigma so that he could self-disclose his condition to certain others, and
- Recognize and use his considerable talents that had not been the focus of the vocational rehabilitation program.

Summary

Depression is a sometimes cyclical, sometimes chronic emotional condition in which a consumer experiences major disruptions to his or her pursuit and maintenance of personal goals. Reviewing the depressed person's natural development of an illness identity can help a consumer integrate the persistence of the mood problem into his or her sense of self while still attending to ultimate goals. In addition to the relationship-based interventions highlighted in chapter 7, two specific empirically based intervention strategies were discussed in this chapter: the cognitive and the interpersonal. In chapter 9, problems commonly experienced by persons diagnosed with bipolar disorder are reviewed.

Major Chapter Learning Points

- While most people experience periods of depression in their lives, major depressive disorder is characterized by chronic or recurring depressive episodes that significantly interfere with a person's ability to function in keeping with his or her primary personal goals.
- Persons with chronic depression tend to move through four stages of illness identity development, an understanding of which can help social workers attend to consumers' nontherapy needs for connection and acceptance.
- Psychosocial interventions that may be helpful for persons with depression include interpersonal therapy, psychodynamic therapy, nondirective supportive treatment, CBT, behavioral activation treatment, and problem-solving therapy.
- Practitioners can be of great assistance to a consumer's family by helping them understand the nature of depression and recovery.

Questions for Reflection or Discussion

1. How can a social worker differentiate the influence of biological and psychological influences on a consumer's depression? How might that be done in the two chapter vignettes?
2. Should the social worker have addressed the physical abuse that characterized Barbara's adult family history in a different way?
3. Could the social worker have done more to help Barbara's husband understand her needs to be active outside the household?
4. Mike had much experience with practitioners, and seemed to have an understanding of what he "should" say, or was expected to say to them. What does this attitude imply about his previous counseling experiences, and how can a social worker ensure that a consumer is honest about his or her goals or lack of them?

Chapter 9

Bipolar Disorder

Bipolar disorder is a disorder of mood in which a person experiences one or more manic episodes that usually alternate with periods of major depression (APA, 2000). Depressive episodes were described in chapter 8. A manic episode is a period in which a person's mood is elevated and expansive to such a degree that he or she experiences serious functional impairment. It is characterized by unrealistically inflated self-esteem, a decreased need for sleep, pressured speech, racing thoughts, distractibility, an increase in unrealistic goal-directed activity, involvement in activities with a high potential for negative consequences, and, sometimes, psychotic symptoms. Manic episodes develop rapidly and may persist for a few days up to several weeks. Another feature associated with bipolar disorder is the hypomanic episode, a gradual escalation from a stable mood to a manic state over a period of days or weeks (APA, 2000). The person experiences mild symptoms of mania, and his or her related behaviors may be socially acceptable, but an eventual escalation into full-blown mania is likely (Grant et al., 2005).

The process of recovery from bipolar disorder is complicated by the fact that it is a recurrent problem. The person may function extremely well when stable, but experience dramatic disruptions in his or her life when manic or depressed. Even with the consistent use of medications, the chances of a person continuing to experience mood cycles are high. For this reason, the process of recovery may not be linear, but may include many starts and stops that can be extremely frustrating and demoralizing. The purpose of this chapter is to describe a range of interventions for social workers to use with consumers who are recovering from bipolar disorder.

There are two types of bipolar disorder (APA, 2000): bipolar I disorder is characterized by one or more manic episodes usually accompanied by a major depressive episode, and bipolar II disorder is characterized by one or more major depressive episodes accompanied by at least one hypomanic episode. While generally milder than bipolar I disorder, bipolar II disorder is characterized by a higher incidence of suicidal ideation (Vieta & Suppes, 2008). For both types of the disorder, the duration between episodes tends to decrease as additional cycles occur (Geller, Tillman, Bolhofner, & Zimerman, 2008).

Prevalence estimates of bipolar disorder range from 0.5 to 5 percent (Matza, Rajagopalan, Thompson, & Lissovoy, 2005). The lifetime prevalence of bipolar I disorder is equal in men and women (close to 1 percent), although bipolar II disorder is more common in women (up to 5 percent) (Barnes & Mitchell, 2005). Between 1994 and 2003, there was a forty-fold increase in child and adolescent diagnoses of the disorder, which may be due to changing diagnostic criteria (presented by various theorists but not adopted by the American Psychiatric Association) or greater practitioner sensitivity to its symptoms (Moreno et al., 2007). Social workers must be extremely cautious in their diagnoses of children, since there is controversy about appropriate criteria with that population (Stone, 2006). Many researchers agree that bipolar disorder can occur in childhood and adolescence, but it presents differently in those age groups (Birmaher et al., 2006). Symptoms that are more specific to childhood include elevated mood, pressured speech, racing thoughts, and hypersensitivity (Youngstrom et al., 2005).

Risk and Resilience Influences

Onset

The etiology of bipolar disorder is primarily biological, although psychological and social stresses are often relevant to the timing of mood episodes (Leahy, 2007). Family history studies indicate a higher-than-average aggregation of bipolar disorder in families. The chances of children with a bipolar parent developing the disorder are between 2 and 10 percent (Youngstrom et al., 2005). Persons who have a first-degree relative with a mood disorder are more likely to have an earlier age of onset than are persons without a familial pattern. Twin studies further support the heritability of the disorder: a study of identical and fraternal twins in which one member of the pair had bipolar disorder showed a concordance rate of 85 percent (McGuffin et al., 2003).

While genetic research remains promising, the core of bipolar disorder remains elusive. The limbic system and its associated regions in the brain are thought to be the primary site of dysfunction for all the mood disorders. Four areas under study include the neurotransmitters, the endocrine system, physical biorhythms, and physical complications during the mother's pregnancy and childbirth (Swann, 2006). Stressful life events play an activating role, especially in early episodes of bipolar disorder, with subsequent episodes often arising with less clear external precipitants (Newman, 2006). Many of these life events are associated with social rhythm disturbances, including sleep, wake, and activity cycles (Berk et al., 2007). Persons with bipolar disorder who have a history of extreme early-life adversity, such as physical or sexual abuse, show an earlier age of onset, faster and more frequent cycling, and more suicidal ideation (Post et al., 2001).

Course and Outcome

Bipolar I disorder is highly recurrent, with 90 percent of persons who have a manic episode developing future episodes (Sierra et al., 2007). The number of episodes tends to average four over ten years. Approximately 50 percent of persons with bipolar disorder move through alternating manic and depressed cycles, and 10 percent experience rapid cycling (Tyrer, 2006). It is estimated that 40 percent have a mixed type of the disorder, in which a prolonged depressive episode features short bursts of mania. Women are at risk for an episode of bipolar disorder in the postpartum stage, and experience rapid cycling more than men do, possibly because of hormonal differences and changes in thyroid function (Barnes & Mitchell, 2005). A majority of persons with bipolar disorder (70 to 90 percent) return to a stable mood and functioning capacity between episodes. Between 5 and 15 percent of persons with bipolar II disorder develop a manic episode within five years, at which point their diagnosis must be changed to bipolar I disorder (APA, 2000). A recent meta-analysis summarized the predictors of relapse in bipolar disorder, including the number of previous episodes, a history of anxiety, and the occurrence of stressful life events (Altman, Haeri, & Cohen, 2006). Other predictors include poor occupational functioning, a lack of social support, and high levels of family conflict.

Persons with bipolar disorder tend to experience serious occupational and social problems (Marangell et al., 2006). One study indicated a stable working capacity in only 45 percent of consumers (Hirschfeld et al., 2003). Missed work, poor work quality, and conflicts with coworkers all contribute to the downward trend for persons who cannot maintain mood stability. An adolescent who develops bipolar disorder may also experience an arrest in psychological development, thus developing self-efficacy problems that endure into adulthood (Floersch, 2003).

Consumers who experience high levels of life stress after the onset of bipolar disorder are more likely to experience relapse than are consumers with low levels of stress (Tyrer, 2006). Events that can cause these episodes include disruptions in social and family supports and changes in daily routines or sleep-wake cycles, such as air travel and changes in work schedules. One study found that relapse risk was related to ongoing harsh comments from relatives (Schenkel et al., 2008).

Consumers who experience any kind of long-term mental disorder often experience stigma, but certain characteristics of bipolar disorder create unique issues related to stigma.

Stigma in Bipolar Disorder

Persons with bipolar disorder often believe, in the aftermath of a manic or depressive episode, that they have ruined their lives. For anyone, building a successful life requires steadiness and focus. The problems generated by bipolar disorder, however, may repeatedly interrupt these processes, and consumers often face the prospect of starting over. They may become demoralized and experience shame and regret, understanding they have done things that resulted in negative consequences for themselves and others. They may indefinitely carry a sense of self-doubt. Social workers must recognize the difficulties consumers face in these contexts, and the ongoing effects of social stigma they are likely to face (Newman, Leahy, Beck, Reilly-Harrington, & Gyulai, 2002). Recovery practitioners must acknowledge the reality of stigma while helping consumers develop the more functional perspective that they must assume responsibility for taking care of their health as best they can. Consumers face the burden of having to be more vigilant about their health than many other people have to be.

It is fortunate when a person finds supportive friends, family, and colleagues after he or she develops bipolar disorder. Even in benign social circles, however, people may tend to judge the consumer, or think of him or her as fragile. These people may be well-meaning family members. Consumers who come to terms with their illness may experience a setback if they perceive that their own relatives feel stigmatized by their presence in the family. This can take the forms of denial or over-interpreting the consumer's behavior as pathological.

The first step in challenging stigma is for consumers to acknowledge their bipolar disorder to themselves. This is not easy, especially early in the course of the illness. Bipolar disorder often features long periods of mood stability, so its ongoing risks may be difficult for consumers to accept. Practitioners must not make the mistake of confronting consumers for not readily accepting intervention because consumers do not resolve those ambivalent feelings quickly. The challenges of stigma and self-disclosure may intensify when the consumer encounters new people who may play significant roles in their lives. Dilemmas about self-disclosure increase consumers' stress levels, which is the very thing they need to avert to reduce the risk of new episodes. Thus, a second step in challenging stigma is for practitioners to help consumers weigh the pros and cons of self-disclosure for each situation and provide support in the aftermath of attempts to share details of the disorder with another person. When properly educated, those other persons may become excellent supports.

Standard Interventions

Medication is always recommended as a primary intervention for bipolar disorder, but psychosocial interventions can be helpful for controlling its course. Service providers generally prefer to first stabilize a consumer's mental status and then introduce psychosocial interventions (Fava, Ruini, & Rafanelli, 2005).

Medications

The Food and Drug Administration (FDA) has approved a number of medications for the treatment of bipolar disorder (Ketter & Wang, 2010). Most physicians recommend that consumers take medication even after their moods stabilize to reduce the risk of recurrence of another mood episode. Generally, a single mood-stabilizing drug is not effective indefinitely, and a combination of medications may be used (Hamrin & Pachler, 2007). Medications are also used with children who have bipolar disorder, although none has been subjected to randomized, controlled trials (Findling, 2009).

Lithium is the best studied of the mood-stabilizing drugs. It stabilizes both manic and depressive episodes, although it takes several weeks to take effect and is more effective for treating manic than mixed or rapid-cycling episodes (Huang, Lei, & El-Mallach, 2007). Another class of medications, the anticonvulsants, is also effective for the treatment of bipolar disorder. Like Lithium, they are not effective in treating mania in its earliest stages, but they usually begin to stabilize a person's mood in two to five days (Melvin et al., 2008). Many doctors prescribe antipsychotic medications on a short-term basis to quickly control the agitation and psychotic symptoms that may accompany consumers' mood episodes. Approximately one-third of persons with bipolar disorder use small doses of these drugs during the maintenance phase of treatment to help contain periods of agitation (Faravelli, Rosi, & Scarpato, 2006).

Psychosocial Interventions

There is no evidence that psychotherapy without medication can eliminate the risk of bipolar disorder in persons with other predisposing factors. However, psychosocial interventions have an important role in educating the consumer about the illness and its repercussions so that it can be controlled (Miklowitz, Otto, & Frank, 2007). Teaching consumers to identify early warning signs of manic or depressive episodes can significantly reduce the frequency of those episodes (Altman et al., 2006). Consumers' feelings and beliefs about their illness greatly affect their medication adherence. In addition, many people with bipolar disorder continue to have problems in their work and social environments despite medication use, and psychosocial intervention can help improve functioning in these areas (Miklowitz & Otto, 2006). Psychosocial interventions can also help people with bipolar disorder develop a regular schedule for daily living activities, such as sleep, meals, exercise, and work, and prevent disrupted rhythms or stressful life events from triggering a bipolar episode.

Empirical support has been found for three types of interventions incorporating the above elements (Miklowitz & Otto, 2006):

1. Interpersonal and social rhythm therapy is based on the assumption that interpersonal conflicts are a major source of depression for consumers, including those with bipolar disorder (Frank, 2007). It also promotes the person's structured scheduling of daily activities.

2. CBT interventions challenge a consumer's cognitions that may activate episodes of mania or depression (such as "I have no control over my moods"), and can also target cognitions related to medication compliance (Basco & Rush, 2005). CBT further incorporates consumer education and systematic problem-solving strategies (Szentagotai & David, 2010).

3. Family-focused therapy helps those persons to develop communication and problem-solving skills that can help in a consumer's recovery. As discussed earlier, negative expressed emotion from significant others is associated with poorer outcomes in bipolar disorder (Miklowitz, Wisniewski, Miyahara, Otto, & Sachs, 2005).

Two examples of recovery practice are presented next. The first of these features a consumer who has accepted the nature of her disorder and been engaged in a lifelong struggle to contain it, while the second example describes a consumer who has always had doubts that she experienced a condition requiring professional intervention.

The Social Worker

Felicia is a twenty-nine-year-old Latina social worker who is devoting her career to working with people who are homeless. She has had, and continues to have, struggles with mental illness, having been diagnosed with bipolar disorder in adolescence. Her recovery journey has been long and arduous, and while she continues to experience severe mood swings, she has come to view them as a learning experience. "Losing your sense of reality to the point where you lose self-control is frightening. Once you come out of the experience, though, and reflect on the event, and recognize it as just one piece of your life, you can learn to prevent or cope with events that lead to its coming back." This vignette is told largely in Felicia's own words and concludes with her excellent recommendations for recovery-oriented social workers. Notice the strengths, especially those related to her academic life, that Felicia draws on as she tries to manage her disruptive mood episodes.

Felicia grew up in a mid-size city in the eastern United States with her parents and two younger siblings, a sister and a brother. Their existence was materially stable, but she experienced frightening sensations and emotions from an early age:

Felicia Speaks

For much of my life, the loss of control I experienced was an outcome of severe depression. As a young child, I internalized all my stress. I was so paranoid and anxious that I rarely spoke in public until my last two years of high school. To me, at that age, all of this seemed normal, but my parents became concerned and got me into therapy as a young adolescent. Therapy has been pretty continuous for me since then. By now I've had six therapists and six psychiatrists.

When one of my first therapists asked if I felt depressed, I said no, because I didn't consider my nightly crying fits to be abnormal. Still, I agreed to try medications, and my life changed quickly, for the better. I came out of my shell and started speaking up at school. At first, everything seemed to be great. Before long I had my first boyfriend. Even though my sleep schedule changed drastically, because I wasn't so tired all the time, I felt rested. I wasn't paranoid anymore of people watching me from behind their cars. My grades remained high—I was always a diligent student—but I remember not having to pretend to be happy anymore. For the first time, I could feel muscles in my face smile. When bad things happened around me, I could cope without withdrawing. I was sad but not depressed when a friend's mother committed suicide, and when a friend from my high school art class hung himself. These were terrible events, but I got through them.

The improvements in my mood didn't last, though. Anxiety got the best of me during my first year of college; I was fifty miles away from home, living in a dormitory. It was horrible, and for the first time I was briefly hospitalized with uncontrollable shaking and suicidal thoughts. I didn't bounce back quickly from this episode, and for months after I left the hospital I felt like a science experiment of pharmaceutical drugs as my psychiatrist changed dosages and tweaked their combinations. I was struggling emotionally, but was able to return to school, make up the exams and assignments I had missed, and move into the spring semester. Through the following year, I worked closely with my psychiatrist and tried one combination of drugs after another in search of the perfect balance with the least annoying side effects. As the meds changed, so did my mood, but for the worse, and my ability to continue school was threatened.

I barely remember my second hospitalization, which happened during my second year of college. It resulted from a mixed episode where I literally slept for three weeks after zipping fast-forward with anxious energy through school assignments and staying out late at night for the first time in my life. This was the first time my psychiatrist confirmed that I was having hallucinations, although I know I saw things as a child that my parents dismissed as products of my imagination. Once again I missed a lot of classes but made up my exams and returned for the following school year.

At this point, both my doctor and my parents became pessimistic about my prognosis. My parents had dealt with my grandfather's severe mental illness many years before and had seen how a variety of treatments, including electroshock, were of little help. Despite his eventual positive response to medication, my grandfather was forced to live in an adult home located several hours away from his family and friends. This was my parent's idea of appropriate treatment for me as well, because it's what they knew. They began looking into group homes on my behalf. My doctor agreed that, with my diagnosis of bipolar disorder, a history of mental illness in my family, three weeks of sleeping at the hospital, and seemingly little success with medications, a group home might be an appropriate placement for me.

I never wanted to settle for that option, but my parents, though they meant well, had long ago established a pattern of wanting to make decisions for me, assuming I didn't have good enough judgment. I resisted their controlling actions and we were in conflict more and more often. My parents second-guess many of my major life decisions, such as wanting to live alone in my own apartment, and they are not shy about interfering. I got along well with my siblings through the years, although we're not as close as I'd like. They had their own friends, and because they never developed symptoms of mental illness, their lives unfolded much differently from mine.

Then, something positive happened during the summer before my third year in college. After all the trouble I'd had, I somehow managed to work successfully at a sandwich shop, dosed up on medications. The regular schedule and repetitive work was just what I needed. I didn't have to think about anything other than making sandwiches all day, and with the responsibility of work I could, with difficulty, get myself out of bed and bathe every morning. Without the job, I probably would have been hospitalized, but my ability to keep the job was enough to convince my parents to put off the group home plans and let me go back to college in the fall. I learned from this experience that structure was very good for me, and that's still true.

Unfortunately, just a few months into my junior year, I was hospitalized for the third time. This one was a result of a planned suicide attempt. Several things brought me to this point. During a manic episode I allowed myself to cheat with my best friend and roommate's boyfriend, whom I didn't even like. We carried on for months, and in the midst of the mania, I moved in with him and a homeless alcoholic man, who ended up stealing my "boyfriend's" credit cards and car. I stupidly believed that my best friend didn't know what her boyfriend and I were doing. Eventually, the alcoholic man became psychotic—he also had bipolar disorder—lost his job, and ended up being institutionalized after I pressed charges against him for forcing me into his car during a psychotic rage. I finally faced reality and admitted that my best friend knew we had been cheating on her. I was left to clean up the mess that the homeless man had made, in addition to attending to the court hearings for the man's competency and abduction charge. This was my lowest point yet. I was humiliated and lost the support of my family and other friends. I had burned all of my bridges.

At this time I was frustrated about the medications not working, had missed classes and dropped out of another semester of school, was having regular panic attacks, and still wasn't being honest with my psychiatrist that my medications weren't working. Furthermore, two weeks after being told that my plans to study abroad would not happen due to my bipolar disorder and ineligibility for insurance coverage, I attempted to overdose on three boxes of various sleeping pills. Of course, true to form, before doing so I made sure to complete my college group projects, say good-bye to my family, and lie to both my psychiatrist and therapist about how I was doing. I was furious when I woke up in a hospital thinking that I couldn't even succeed at killing myself!

As I've said, up to that point I had never been honest with my therapists or psychiatrists. I never disclosed to my therapists how troubled I was, or the extent of symptoms I was experiencing, because I was in denial. That may seem odd, because I knew I had serious problems, but I was trying to minimize them for myself, and if I was open with my therapists I would have to admit them to myself, too. My therapists were decent people, but looking back I think they always made me feel abnormal, probably because they followed the medical, disease model of mental illness and never looked at me as a total person, I think. It takes an extremely affirming, empathic therapist to help a person get past this desire to minimize a serious problem, and I didn't have that experience until relatively recently. I kept agreeing to try different kinds of medications because I wanted to feel normal again, if only by chemical means. I had all sorts of side effects, but I didn't want to say too much about those because I was afraid the doctors would take me off the medications and then I'd feel my symptoms more strongly. And I wanted to feel normal!

One of the big challenges of bipolar disorder is that a person has to make a decision at some point about the costs and benefits of stabilization. I never felt comfortable taking medication, partly because it caused me to lose important parts of my identity. I have always been an artist, sketching and painting, but when I took medications I couldn't produce anything. Medications helped stabilize my mood to some degree, but they also took something away from me. I was ambivalent about stabilizing, because there are good things about being manic and hypomanic. I feel alive and I'm productive with my art. But, for me, I had to hit rock bottom, to have an experience where I lost everything that was dear to me, to understand that stabilization was worth whatever costs it included. Now I'm committed to keeping myself stable as well as I can.

I had another hospitalization during my final year of college, and it was at that time, for some reason, I became a self-advocate rather than a passive treatment recipient. For the first time, I resisted my parents' desires to place me in a supervised living environment. In fact, we became estranged at that point. Fortunately, I got involved at that time with the first therapist who was actually a positive influence in my recovery. She treated me as if I was a normal person in spite of my emotional difficulties, and her acceptance made a powerful impression on me. I don't remember anything specific she said, but her attitude conveyed the message, "You'll get through this!" She said it in ways that were sincere, and I believed her. She encouraged me to network with people who had the same challenges I did, and she introduced me to a woman who was to become my best friend. I couldn't continue working with that therapist because of moving on to graduate school, but I was fortunate to meet another therapist on the new campus who also gave me hope that I had strengths and could overcome my mood problems.

All this time I was not familiar with a recovery philosophy of mental illness. I tended to think of myself in a defensive way, as always being at risk for falling apart emotionally. I'd had a long list of professionals in my life, but I finally met two social workers who seemed interested in what I could achieve, not merely in how I could avoid failing. This was most fortunate, and a major turning point in my life. I don't think these thera-pists were trained in recovery practice, but they had a natural empathy that embodied the best of the recovery philosophy. They seemed to care about me as a person, and helped me understand that I could learn from my negative experiences, make the most of the capabilities I had, and make changes in my behavior to have different outcomes in my life. I developed a perspective that my life journey was itself the destination, not merely the way to get there, wherever that would be.

I became involved in the recovery movement shortly after beginning my graduate program in social work. I had tried attending a variety of support groups before then, but didn't like them much. Most everyone was much older than me, and they seemed to like complaining more than taking action to make themselves better people. I know I have to respect where anyone else is with his or her recovery processes, but those groups weren't for me. Through an acquaintance, I learned about some-thing called The Icarus Project and investigated it online.

The Icarus Project is a web-based network of people affected by experiences that are labeled as mental illnesses. It promotes a culture that affirms the perspectives of those per-sons rather than trying to fit their lives into a conventional framework. It consists of a national organizing collective and network of local and campus groups. The collective serves local groups by facilitating a website community, distributing publi-cations, educating the public, engaging in advocacy activities, and providing a sense of solidarity.

Being disappointed with the support groups I had attended, I decided to start my own group, and I registered it online with Icarus. We met every two weeks at different clinics that agreed to provide us with space. My group had a struc-tured format, including icebreakers and art projects, so that participants would be drawn in. It was a great experience for me, and to my surprise many of the participants who regularly attended were mental health professionals with emotional problems of their own. I met many of the principal recovery advocates in my region. The group went on for two years, but I was becoming busier in my personal and work life, and so I passed it on to another leader.

At the present time I am a full-time social worker providing services to my city's homeless population. I don't know that my own life experiences have led me into this kind of work but it's certainly possible. As I experienced ups and downs, I took what I learned to help myself move on to where I wanted to be. I still have regular challenges with my daily rhythms and moods, but I attend to them with the help of some close friends. There are no guarantees for the future, but I am confident that I have learned so much, and with the support of my close friends I will continue to grow.

I'm often asked about my spirituality and how it may have been influenced by my experiences with bipolar disorder. Well, I do believe in God, but more as an ultimate spirit than a being. I really don't know how my spirituality has been influenced by my life experiences. I've always been a lover of art, and believe that art is a transcendent experience that brings people together, but I might have felt the same way without my ups and downs.

One thing I struggle with as a professional is the issue of self-disclosure. I think there is quite a bit of discrimination, even in the mental health community, about practitioners with certain problems. There is also discomfort involved in policing one's colleagues, but social workers do have a responsibility to consumers and to the field as a whole to monitor the activities of their peers who may not be functioning well. Still, it can be discriminatory to judge practitioners who are working effectively, simply because they struggle with bipolar disorder. For example, I don't necessarily want to become a licensed social worker in my state because I would be required to report any future psychiatric hospitalizations and be approved by the board before returning to work. I believe that social workers with bipolar disorder need to monitor themselves and should regularly consult with at least one other professional for therapy and medication.

Felicia's Commentary

The recovery perspective is empowering for persons who have bipolar disorder. Based on my own experiences, I've developed the following recommendations for social workers who work with these consumers:

- Accept the consumer unconditionally, without judgment, disapproval, or approval, at his or her highest and lowest points. The social worker should not be surprised when consumers do unhealthy or surprisingly uncharacteristic things for which others have judged them or broken ties. An empathic and respectful understanding of the consumer allows trust to develop.

- Treat the condition as a challenge, not a disease. Normalizing bipolar disorder allows the consumer to recognize that everyone has challenges, some greater than others, and they are not alone or weird. Recovery is nonlinear, but is based on a continual growth pattern. Encourage a community of supportive peers with similar diagnoses.

- Help the consumer weigh the pros and cons of maintaining stability. Recognize that the highs of mania can be rewarding as well as debilitating.

- Help the consumer reflect on lessons learned from prior mood episodes by creating an individualized action plan. Help the consumer create a concrete list of triggers that can contribute to lapses into mania and depression. As soon as the consumer is able to identify triggers and take responsibility for recovery, he or she can begin to take control over his or her own symptoms and cycles.

- Encourage the consumer to work closely with a psychiatrist to find the right medications, and to be patient. Many drugs have side effects that don't have to be tolerated, and everyone responds to meds differently. Tapering on and off meds can take time and cause instability. Showing consumers you have hope that the right medications can be found will give them hope.

- Be concrete with consumers. Speaking abstractly or philosophizing can sometimes overwhelm and confuse depressed people.

- Repetitive tasks, jobs, and schedules can be therapeutic for consumers experiencing depression. When a consumer is depressed or overwhelmed, help him or her make a daily schedule including activities and times for each day. This should include three to five tasks for each day and include specific eating and sleeping times. Remember that showering and eating can be huge tasks for depressed consumers. Make things simple.

- During conversations with depressed consumers, do not bombard them with questions. This comes across as irritating and frustrating. Instead, talk to the consumer about general and even lighthearted topics. Allow the consumer to listen to the positive thoughts of someone who accepts them in their shutdown state.

- Remember that as a mental health professional you often see the consumers at their worst and most vulnerable state. Do not let this fool you into having low expectations of the consumer. Having a strengths-based perspective will allow the person to build on his or her skills and talents. The consumer must take on the responsibility of living his or her own life and learn to maintain recovery in his or her own way. Having higher expectations of the consumer will allow him or her to achieve more.

The following vignette describes recovery work with a consumer diagnosed with bipolar disorder who never fully committed to a professional intervention process, and never fully accepted that she had a disorder. The practitioner's dilemma is that she believed the consumer's recovery would be facilitated by certain actions that the consumer did not want to take. The social worker was thus tested in her usual desire to be collaborative. Unlike the other vignettes in this book, this is written as a session-by-session narrative to illustrate more deliberately the efforts of the social worker to engage the consumer in a recovery process, with mixed results.

The Interior Designer

Gloria Lee was a fifty-one-year-old African American female, unemployed and living with her ex-husband, who had recently reenrolled in college. She walked into the crisis center one day and insisted on seeing a counselor because of, as she put it, "feeling scared." She reported that the last time she felt this way she became suicidal. Gloria complained of anxiety, depression, unpredictable moods, irritability, an inability to concentrate, and trouble organizing her thoughts. She had felt this way for a few weeks and added, "It happens a lot." After meeting with a crisis intervention worker for forty-five minutes, Gloria relaxed and said she felt better. She was invited back for a formal intake session the next day.

Session #1

At her intake session with the social worker, Allie, Gloria reported the same symptoms as the previous day, adding that she was having trouble paying attention in class. She said "a million thoughts" raced through her head all day long, and they made her feel confused, anxious, and overwhelmed. She reported irritability, an accelerated pace of speech, and an inability to sleep without medicine. Gloria was dealing with a number of stressors: she had come back to school after a long break, recently moved to a new apartment, had had abdominal surgery, lost her job at a restaurant where she had worked for two years, and had no car.

Gloria had five adult stepchildren, a twenty-seven-year-old biological daughter from a previous relationship, and two young grandchildren. She had her biological daughter when she was twenty-four years old but never married the father. She had been married twice, first in 1983 for eight years, and again for about six years beginning in 2000. Gloria reported a great relationship with her second ex-husband, with whom she now lived. Gloria was an older undergraduate student in the local art school, pursuing a major in interior design. She recently had learned that her unmarried daughter was pregnant for the third time, which caused her a great deal of anxiety. She'd had "a few drinks" several times since she learned of the pregnancy and was worried she might start drinking excessively again.

Gloria had been diagnosed about twenty years before with bipolar I disorder, most recent episode manic; alcohol abuse; and generalized anxiety disorder. She reported a lengthy history of psychiatric treatment and three suicide attempts. The onset of her difficulties was about twenty-five years ago. She experienced a number of major stressors around that time related to moving from the West to the East coast. Shortly afterward, she lost a job, was convicted of her first DUI (followed by mandatory participation in a thirty-day inpatient substance abuse program), and was sentenced to six months in prison for a separate charge of breaking and entering. She started to drink heavily and to talk obsessively; she was hospitalized twice, for a few days each time, in a psychiatric facility.

Gloria reported she was first diagnosed with depression, and a few years later with bipolar disorder. At that time she took antidepressant medication for one year but eventually experienced troubling adverse effects, feeling more depressed and having auditory hallucinations, which led to her first suicide attempt. She discontinued the medication and soon felt better. Gloria reported that since this first major breakdown she had had two other DUI convictions and two more suicide attempts (at ages thirty-three and forty). Each suicide attempt occurred during periods of extreme stress and when she was intoxicated. In addition to her psychiatric problems, Gloria had a number of medical illnesses. She had been diagnosed three years before with a chronic lung disease for which she was on medication. The onset of this disease coincided with the time she started college; she had to discontinue school to take care of her health. In addition to medication for her lung disease, Gloria took sleep medication as needed.

Gloria stated that she was always shy by nature and had limited social support, only interacting regularly with her ex-husband and daughter. She felt anxious in social situations and worried that people would think critically of her, or that she might say or do something to embarrass herself. She said she would like to have more friends and was interested in learning to cope with what she called her "social anxiety."

With regard to goals, Gloria reported that she was interested in understanding "what was wrong and how to fix it." She seemed motivated to pursue professional intervention so that she did not have to "deal with the burden of figuring it all out" by herself. Gloria hoped that intervention would be helpful in her learning to manage and stabilize her mood and anxiety, improve her concentration, and develop problem-solving and social skills. She was reluctant to begin taking psychotropic medications but was agreeable to a medication evaluation. She did not believe she was dependent on alcohol since she believed she could stop anytime.

During this first session, Gloria had initially been tense but later presented as relaxed, comfortable, and open, and engaged easily in conversation with the social worker. Her speech was coherent but fast-paced; she admitted that she sometimes stumbled over words trying to keep up with the thoughts in her head. Gloria frequently said that she was relieved to have found someone to talk to. Allie concluded the session by thanking Gloria for providing her personal history and promised that they would begin focusing more on her goals during their next meeting.

Session #2

Allie had planned to begin this session with an overview of her recovery practice philosophy, but as usual she encouraged the consumer to begin the conversation. It quickly became apparent that Gloria was not in the mood for an orientation to the intervention process because she was so upset. Gloria shared her panic about receiving an "F" in one of her courses. She planned to appeal the grade, claiming medical problems, so that she could maintain her active student status. Gloria was upset and tearful as she talked, although she eventually calmed down. She reported that she had been anxious all week about her academic concerns because the university was closed and there was nothing she could do about them until the following week. Gloria admitted to becoming physically ill when anxious and stated she had gone to see a physician twice in the past few weeks about intestinal concerns. She had not yet seen a doctor for a medication evaluation related to her bipolar disorder, but had an appointment for the following week.

Allie was surprised at Gloria's level of anxiety, but willingly focused on her presenting concern. She listened, affirmed the consumer's stress level, and helped her to problem solve in a thoughtful way as an alternative to being immobilized by anxiety. Gloria once again settled down with the social worker's calm approach, and agreed with Allie's suggested plan for appealing the grade. Allie, who knew well how the college operated, spent most of the second half of the meeting helping the consumer articulate and write down the plan of action. Near the end of the session, they talked more generally about the consumer's primary goals for recovery. Gloria's vision was to maintain her current range of activities but develop more social supports so that she would have more people to rely on in times of stress. Gloria was aware that she became overwhelmed by stress and emphasized her desire to develop self-control in this regard. Allie spoke with the consumer about her psychiatric diagnosis and learned that she had little understanding of the nature of her mood swings. Allie suggested that Gloria could indeed manage herself more effectively, and that understanding the nature of her disorder would help her to do so.

When the session was over, Allie thought about the fact that Gloria had, through two visits, been upset at the beginning but settled down once she had an opportunity to vent. Allie was aware that she had primarily been providing Gloria with crisis intervention, which seemed appropriate, but she was also frustrated that she had not yet been able to articulate the desired collaborative nature of their work together, and her other recovery-oriented guiding principles. Allie hoped that the consumer would be as agreeable to coming to meetings when things were going more smoothly for her.

Session #3

Gloria was much calmer this week after having resolved the academic issue to her satisfaction. Her "F" had been changed to an incomplete; she could make up the missed work and receive another grade. She expressed her appreciation of Allie's help in managing this challenge. Gloria had also seen a psychiatrist and begun taking Lithium. With her life now under control, the consumer felt more confident about achieving her goal of better social functioning through greater social support.

With this initial success, and Gloria's calmer demeanor, Allie offered her thoughts about the consumer's strengths and her potential to learn to manage her bipolar disorder and associated challenges more effectively. Gloria admitted again that she did not really know much about bipolar disorder and was suspicious of what she called the "poisonous" effects of the medications. She added that the idea of bipolar disorder "scared [her] to death, because the term is so frightening and [she] liked to think of [herself] as normal." Gloria admitted that the doctor had not spoken to her about Lithium and its purposes.

Allie perceived that Gloria was sensitive to the stigma of mental illness, and from that point on referred to her symptoms as "problems in living," minimizing her use of professional terms. Allie did refer to the consumer's symptoms at times as representing a medical problem, since that made sense to Gloria. The social worker provided Gloria with information about the actions of the drug and its positive and potentially adverse effects. Gloria listened but soon shifted the topic to her desire for more pleasant social interactions and how she might practice with her classmates. Gloria felt awkward in her classes because of her age, a common experience for older students, but Allie discovered that she did have a few same-age classmates. While this conversation was helpful, it seemed to the social worker that Gloria became quite anxious when the topic of her mood disorder was raised. Allie was determined to collaborate with Gloria on her primary goals but thought it might be harmful in the long run to avoid addressing the nature of her disorder.

Session #4

Gloria was pleasant at the beginning of the session but soon became tearful as she recounted a disappointing medical appointment earlier that morning. She had felt disrespected by the physician and nurse, who had asked her to cut back on her smoking and drinking. While Allie empathized with the consumer, she was discovering for the first time how sensitive

Gloria was to perceived criticism and how readily she internalized negative perceptions. Allie asked her about this sensitivity. Gloria tearfully shared her lifelong history of being criticized by others, going back to her family of origin. Allie saw this tendency as a significant issue to address, something that went beyond her experience of bipolar disorder; she perceived that it was a contributing factor to her mood swings. She explained to the consumer that such strongly held biases were known as negative cognitive assumptions and that she might benefit from working on adjusting her arbitrary assumptions. This seemed to make sense to Gloria, although Allie perceived that the consumer was ambivalent about discussing the issue. Gloria seemed threatened by the idea that she had more psychological problems.

Session #5

Gloria was more composed during this session. She reported enjoying school, keeping busy with her studies, visiting with her daughter, and trying to get hold of her physician about a medication issue. Allie praised Gloria for organizing her time in such a productive manner, and she emphasized the importance of structure in Gloria's daily life. Gloria appeared to be an organized person by nature, but she had not been educated about the importance of structure to maintaining mood stability. Her mood on this day was stable and her thought processes clear. It was evident to Allie that there was a close association between Gloria's anxiety and her tendencies to experience mood swings. Furthermore, Gloria seemed to experience distress when she focused on other people to the extent of ignoring her own needs. Allie shared these observations with the consumer, who agreed but again seemed to feel threatened by the idea of her fragility. Allie was always alert to the consumer's reactions to information and was careful to frame it in a positive manner, reminding Gloria that she was functioning well. Allie suggested that they continue focusing on how Gloria could manage stress. The only concern Gloria expressed was that she was becoming concerned about weight gain since starting the Lithium.

It was during this and the following two sessions that Allie and Gloria focused most systematically on the consumer's recovery process. Gloria had learned that lifestyle changes, including adhering to a schedule, would help her realize her goals of satisfactory social functioning through increased social support. It was also clear, however, that the consumer was becoming skeptical again about taking medications and was not sure that she had a mental disorder. Allie had continued to focus on Gloria's strengths but also monitored her symptoms. The consumer admitted she had a hard time accepting that she had a mental disorder because the idea frightened her. Allie responded that no matter how Gloria thought about her problems, she could take charge of her own well-being.

Session #6

Gloria was pleasant and calm. She had seen her psychiatrist and general practitioner during the past week for monitoring of her mental health and medical concerns. Allie praised her for responsibly attending to these tasks and expressing her concerns about medications to both persons. Gloria was feeling good physically and about herself in general. When Allie asked about her progress toward her goals, she maintained that it was positive, although it did not appear that Gloria was actively working to expand her range of social supports. Gloria added that she wanted to add regular exercise and better nutrition to her list of goals, so they discussed ways for her to introduce these activities into her day.

Session #7

This session appeared to Allie to represent a peak of Gloria's recovery. She looked healthy and said she had enjoyed optimistic attitudes most of the week. She had come to feel comfortable with her medication regimen and was not presently concerned about weight gain and other side effects. Furthermore, the consumer was developing a stronger sense of self that did not require her to suit the expectations of others. Allie observed that the consumer appeared to be doing well but she was curious to learn how Gloria would respond the next time a significant problem arose. Perhaps her coping capacity was improving. Gloria was continuing to manage her daily routines well, avoid unmanageable stress, and take medications as prescribed, with apparent positive effect. She responded well to Allie's support and encouragement to monitor her moods, and was organizing her time constructively. Allie was concerned that Gloria was still limiting her interactions to her ex-husband and daughter, but could not deny that the consumer was doing well. Gloria stated that she would like to begin coming in every two weeks from this point, given that she was feeling stable and capable of self-direction.

Session #8

It was in this session that Gloria's quality of functioning went into decline, precipitated by new stressors. The consumer had experienced major disruptions in her social routines due to her daughter's giving birth to her third child. Gloria was being called upon to help her daughter adjust to this event and was happy to oblige, but was again missing sleep and classes. Gloria's anxiety was increasing, and she expressed new concerns about possible side effects of her medication. Allie was concerned that Gloria was now more susceptible to mood swings and reminded her of the importance of taking her own needs into account as well as those of her daughter. Gloria agreed, but in fact seemed to discount the importance of self-care, because she didn't want to let her daughter down. In spite of these threatening developments, Gloria appeared to be exercising good judgment and managing herself fairly well. Allie reminded the consumer to persist with taking care of her student demands and medical issues, and Gloria seemed responsive to those prompts.

Session #9

Gloria returned to the agency after a difficult few weeks that included receiving an eviction notice from her apartment for nonpayment of rent, a mugging in which she was not seriously hurt but was traumatized and had her purse stolen, and difficulties completing her coursework. Still, she and her ex-husband appeared to have weathered these events well and were excited about moving into a new rental unit. Gloria did describe what she perceived to be more discomforting adverse effects from her medication, and said she had stopped taking it, although she promised to see her psychiatrist the following week about this. She said she was "anxious but not overwhelmed." Allie was concerned again, however, by the consumer's tendency to minimize her health problems and her own goals when external challenges emerged. They talked at length about the consumer's decision to stop taking medication; Gloria was adamant that she did not want to resume it.

The Phone Calls

Gloria missed her next scheduled appointment, and Allie was not able to reach her for another week. When they finally spoke by phone, Gloria said she had been in the hospital for physical problems unrelated to her psychiatric condition. She had missed her psychiatrist appointment and had been off Lithium for a month now. She reported, too, the tragic news that her infant granddaughter had died unexpectedly. Gloria was spending a lot of time supporting her daughter through this crisis. As a result of these incidents, the consumer had not been able to, or had not wanted to, come to the agency, although she confirmed she would do so once her family issues settled down. Allie strongly encouraged Gloria to contact her at that time. In fact, she encouraged Gloria to call whenever she wanted to talk.

Allie spoke with the consumer by phone several more times during the next month. Gloria had called for an appointment because of a personal crisis related to her ex-husband's plans to move away and leave her alone. They had experienced major conflicts about the role of her daughter in their lives; the ex-husband felt that Gloria was making her daughter a priority above all else. Although Gloria seemed distressed during the call, she later cancelled the appointment due to her need to, as she said, "take care of some money issues." It seemed again that Gloria was not attending to her own needs, and was being sidetracked by external events. Allie was not sure if Gloria would come to the agency again but left the door open for her to do so. Gloria never did come back, calling twice during the next four months for appointments but never following through.

One Year Later

Gloria contacted the agency director (not Allie) by phone. She did not introduce herself, but said she "saw a number come up on [my] cell phone and just pushed it." She was calling from New Orleans, where she was visiting a niece, and said she was planning to return to Virginia in a week or so. She said she had seen Allie more than a year ago but had not continued due to medical problems. In a tone the director described as "rapid and giddy," Gloria asked the agency director to give Allie the message that she would like to speak to her. When the director asked if there was anything Gloria wanted her to tell Allie, she responded, "Tell Allie I'm still here, and I'll be back soon." That was Gloria's final contact with the agency.

Commentary   Allie, in her own view, had limited success in helping Gloria move through a recovery process with her bipolar disorder and anxiety. The practitioner reviewed her work with the consumer after the consumer dropped out of intervention, and identified the following possible obstacles to Gloria's recovery:

- Gloria had a crisis orientation to counseling, and was only open to receiving help when she was in active distress over some issue. Allie wondered if she might have done a better job helping Gloria see the bigger picture of the impact of mood swings on her overall life in a context of her strengths and limitations.
- Gloria had physical problems, and tended to attribute her emotional problems to those.
- Gloria was reluctant to invest in a sustained intervention process. She never seemed to consider the possible value of sustained regular recovery work in developing a suitable lifestyle.
- Gloria had difficulty accepting that she had a disorder, in part due to her self-imposed sense of stigma. Although Allie had worked hard not to frame the consumer's problems as related to a disorder, the client was getting that message from others and was sensitive to the associated stigma. Gloria believed, possibly accurately, that her family would not accept her as a normal person if

she spoke to them about this. Allie might have addressed the issue of stigma more directly.

Gloria's situation was indicative, to Allie, of a paradox of recovery intervention for some persons, in that a degree of awareness of having a disorder may sometimes be necessary to move beyond it. Another lesson to be learned from this illustration is that relationship factors do not always make for an atmosphere of disclosure. Allie did her best to be patient, supportive, and collaborative with Gloria, but this was not sufficient to help the consumer through her tendency to minimize her emotional needs.

In summary, however, it is possible that this intervention was significant to Gloria's recovery process. Gloria did remember Allie and called her a year later. All persons move through recovery at their own pace, and it is possible that Gloria experienced learning in her work with Allie that might help her be more open to further recovery-focused intervention in the future.

Summary

Bipolar disorder is a disorder of mood associated with certain unstable nervous system processes. The disorder may present consumers with a host of problems related to self-image and psychosocial functioning that can be addressed with recovery-based intervention. Whether or not consumers understand the condition to be biological, social workers can help them organize their lives in such a way that they may acquire greater levels of self-confidence and personal mastery, and thus achieve and maintain their goals. A challenge to recovery intervention with bipolar clients is addressing their occasional periods of poor judgment that may be evident during the active phases of the disorder. The social worker may feel compelled to take over intervention initiatives, as described in the second illustration, to prevent the client from experiencing potentially devastating symptoms.

Major Chapter Learning Points

- Bipolar disorder is a disorder of mood in which a person experiences one or more manic episodes that usually alternate with periods of depression. A manic episode is a period in which a person's mood is elevated to such a degree that he or she experiences functional impairment in all areas of life.

- The process of recovery from bipolar disorder is complicated by the fact that it is a recurrent problem. The person may function extremely well when stable, but experience dramatic disruptions in his or her life when manic or depressed.
- Bipolar disorder is considered to be biological in origin, although psychosocial factors may affect its course.
- Stigma, whether societal or self-generated, may be particularly acute with bipolar disorder, since the person functions well when stable and thus may minimize the significance of the disorder. Consumers benefit from acknowledging the disorder to themselves, and then considering disclosure to certain significant others.

Questions for Reflection or Discussion

1. This issue came up earlier in the book, but how can a recovery practitioner interact with a client like Felicia to minimize her lying to him or her?
2. Felicia described herself as experiencing "uncontrollable shaking and suicidal thoughts" during her first year of college, which led to her first hospitalization. How might a recovery-focused practitioner work with a consumer to initiate such a hospitalization while staying true to the recovery principle of self-direction?
3. How might a practitioner inadvertently overlook any of the recommendations in Felicia's commentary?
4. How might Allie have helped Gloria gain some perspective and take a holistic view of her strengths and limitations as a step toward assuming more power over her life?
5. How might Allie have more thoroughly addressed the issue of Gloria's stigma?
6. Would you consider Allie's intervention with Gloria to be successful in helping the consumer begin to recover from her mental illness? Why or why not?

Chapter 10

The Autism Spectrum Disorders

Joseph Walsh, Amy Wagner, and Brittany Leggett

Three related disorders comprise the autism spectrum disorders (ASD): autism, Asperger's disorder, and pervasive developmental disorder not otherwise specified (PDD-NOS). These all begin in childhood and are characterized by "severe and pervasive impairment in several areas of development: reciprocal social interaction, communication skills, or the presence of stereotyped behavior, interests, and activities" (APA, 2000, p. 65). Autism is the best known of these disorders, but researchers speculate that the ASD may represent different levels of the same core disorder. The ASD have been increasingly diagnosed in recent years, and because they require such intensive intervention, often with modest impact, they represent a major challenge to the health-care professions.

The purpose of this chapter is to discuss how recovery practice can be implemented with a consumer population that often is not able to articulate its own goals or participate collaboratively with intervention. Of course, the caregivers of persons with ASD usually assume active roles in the intervention process. Social work recovery practice with ASD consumers almost always involves advocacy activities on their, and the family's, behalf, toward the development of social resources that can best accommodate their needs.

Autism is characterized by abnormal development in social interaction and communication, and a stereotypical, repetitive range of behaviors such as rocking, toe-walking, flapping, clapping, whirling, and an obsessive desire for sameness (Schreibman, Stahmer, & Akshoomoff, 2006). Despite differences in presentation, impairments in social relatedness always underlie the disorder (Volkmar, Chwarska, & Klin, 2005). These include a lack of awareness of the feelings of others, an impaired capacity to imitate and express emotion, and the absence of a capacity for social play. Even in infancy, children with autism may lack a capacity for reciprocal social engagement. As the child grows older, these social disabilities persist. Communication deficits in persons with autism include a reliance on nonverbal communication; repetition of words or phrases; atypical speech rhythm, intonation, and loudness; and pronoun reversal (Akshoomoff, 2006). Persons with autism may present irrelevant details, inappropriately perseverate on a topic, suddenly shift to a new topic, and ignore others' attempts to initiate conversation. Deficits also involve language comprehension: these persons interpret speech in overly concrete ways. Persons with autism do, however, often possess pockets of ability, such as memorization, visual and spatial skills, and attention to details.

As noted earlier, in the past twenty years researchers have observed that the characteristics of autism are spread across the two other spectrum disorders without clear lines of demarcation among them. The core symptoms of autism are less severe in these other two diagnostic categories. In Asperger's disorder, the early development of cognition and language is apparently normal, but the child often has unusual interests that are pursued with great intensity (Holter, 2004). The child's approaches to peers and new adults may be idiosyncratic, but attachment patterns to family members are well established. Social deficits become more prominent as the child enters school and is exposed to peers. Persons with this condition generally have a better outcome than those with autism—they are more likely to attain employment, live independently, and establish a family (Howlin, 2005). Still, the social difficulties of Asperger's disorder are lifelong. PDD-NOS encompasses a subthreshold form of autism in which there is marked impairment in social interaction, communication, or behavior patterns or interests, but the full features of the other two diagnoses are not met (Koyama, Tachimor, & Osada, 2006). This category is, fortunately, more commonly diagnosed than the other two, and represents the highest level of functioning within the ASD spectrum, but its related problems may be prominent during the school years.

Autism does not appear later than the age of three and is usually diagnosed by age four or five (Smith, Magyar, & Arnold-Saritepe, 2002). The other spectrum disorders may not be diagnosed until several years later because their symptoms are not as prominent. In the first year of life, the child with an ASD displays unusual social development, is less likely to imitate the movements and vocal sounds of others, and exhibits problems with attention and responding to external stimulation (Volkmar et al., 2005). Between ages one to three years, when parents are most likely to seek evaluation, differences from peers are readily apparent, and the person's self-absorbed behaviors and communication problems are striking.

The reported incidence of the ASD has increased at a high rate in the past twenty years. The causes of this increase include changing diagnostic criteria, service eligibility regulations, knowledge about effective interventions, and political advocacy (Shattuck & Grosse, 2007). The Centers for Disease Control and Prevention (CDC, 2012) stated that, as of 2012, the prevalence of the ASD is 11.3 per 1,000 children in the United States.

The disorders occur more often in males than females, with a 4.3 to 1 ratio, but there are no social class or ethnic differences in prevalence (Liptak, Stuart, & Auinger, 2006). Persons with ASD experience a high range of co-occurring disorders due to their broadly debilitating features, associated medical conditions, and the problematic life experiences related to having them (de Bruin, Ferdinand, Meester, de Nijs, & Verheij, 2007). Common co-occurring disorders include mental retardation, seizure disorders, depression, and anxiety.

A Recovery Focus with the ASD

The growth in identified cases of ASD, and the financial expense of comprehensive intervention, has created a situation where many such children do not receive adequate medical, educational, and behavioral health care for achieving their highest functioning potential. The needs of persons with an ASD place health-care providers and insurers at a high financial risk. The mean total annual expenditures of children with ASD in 2006 was $6,132, of which 65 percent went for outpatient expenses and of which only 10 percent was paid out of pocket (Liptak et al., 2006). Much of this spending went to home health care, including care attendants and home-based workers. By contrast, children without ASD only generated an average of $860 in annual health-care costs. Children with ASD carry a substantial burden of medical care, averaging 42 outpatient visits (versus 3.3 for other children) and twenty-two prescription medications and refills per year; 24 percent of children with an ASD take psychotropic medications.

Federal law mandates the provision of an appropriate educational plan for all children with ASD in the United States (Holter, 2004). As part of this plan, ancillary services are often required, including speech or language therapy, occupational therapy, and physical therapy. Sustained, continuous programming is more effective than episodic programming; summer programming is also recommended because children with ASD often regress in the absence of such services.

Medicaid is the largest single public payer of behavioral health services, and accounts for 75 percent of all funding for developmentally disabled related services (Beasley & Hurley, 2007). Because children with disabilities consume more services than those without disabilities, financial incentives to control costs have a greater impact on them. A study of service use by persons with ASD in one state's (Tennessee) Medicaid managed care program illustrates the effects of public funding on the problem (Ruble, Heflinger, Renfrew, & Saunders, 2005). The major finding of this study was that although the number of children who received services increased, that number represented only one-tenth of the estimated number of persons with ASD. While more costly services such as day treatment disappeared, case management and medication management services increased. Cost shifting to other service sectors such as schools added an additional source of diffusion of responsibility.

Another major issue for public policy is what will happen when the large numbers of children with ASD become adults and leave the school systems, the primary public institutions for their service delivery. When these persons reach age eighteen, many will quality for Supplemental Security Insurance and Medicaid. Currently, people with disabilities comprise 15 percent of all Medicaid recipients but account for 37 percent of expenditures (Flanders, Engelhart, Pandina, & McCracken, 2007). The long-term care components of these expenditures will rise significantly if the ASD population of tomorrow requires the same levels of care as today's population.

The recovery philosophy of intervention incorporates a central belief that the experience of people with a disability, rather than the expertise of professionals, should be the critical factor in policy making (Reindal, 2008). This approach emphasizes both self-advocacy and professional advocacy, and a resolve that the world should be altered to accommodate persons with disabilities, rather than altering the people who have those disabilities. Since the recovery philosophy suggests in part that autism is not a disabling condition per se, but that the problem lies in how society treats people with autism, a case can be made that fewer resources should be devoted to eradicating ASD, and more resources should be devoted to understanding and addressing the specific needs of those persons. Parents of such children should be able to think about what interventions they need, and a combination of public and private resources might ensure greater access to those services. At the same time, society should begin to understand the need to embrace all marginalized individuals, including those with autism.

Risk and Resilience Influences

Onset

The ASD are genetic, neurobiological disorders (Maimberg & Vaeth, 2006). There is no association of ASD with any psychological influences, including parenting styles. Although many parents believe that vaccinations are the cause of the ASD (Harrington, Rosen, Garnecho, & Patrick, 2006), the Institute of Medicine (2004) has determined that no such links have been established. Approximately 60 to 70 percent of persons with ASD manifest distinct neurological abnormalities and various levels of mental retardation. Brain abnormalities exist in a majority of diagnosed individuals, but 30 to 40 percent of persons with ASD possess an anatomically intact central nervous system (Peliosa & Lund, 2001). Thus, ASD appears to have many etiologies, including

- Genetic conditions,
- Viral infections (such as congenital rubella, a type of mental retardation that results from infection during pregnancy),
- Metabolic conditions (such as abnormalities of purine, the amino acid that energizes many physical reactions), and
- Congenital anomaly syndromes (such as Williams' syndrome, a genetic disability characterized by outgoing behavior and intellectual and developmental deficits).

Course and Adjustment

Studies on the course of ASD show variable outcomes that depend on the severity of the condition. Several studies have been conducted in

Sweden. In one study, children who had been diagnosed with ASD (N = 120) were assessed in adulthood (Billstedt, Gillberg, & Gillberg, 2005). The majority (57 percent) was categorized as having a "very poor" outcome. The next common outcome was "poor" (21 percent), followed by "restricted" (13 percent), and "fair" (8 percent). None of the persons had a "good" outcome. In another study, Swedish men diagnosed with autism or Asperger's disorder were followed for five years after diagnosis (Cederlund, Hagberg, Billstedt, Gillberg, & Gillberg, 2008). In the majority of cases of persons with Asperger's disorder, the diagnosis was still valid (84 percent), and even those without the ongoing diagnosis showed impairment. About 25 percent of the Asperger's sample had a poor outcome, despite having average IQs. Outcomes were less promising for the persons in the autism group, with the majority (76 percent) having "poor" to "very poor" outcomes. Intellectual levels were lower among those in the autism group, where only five (7 percent) persons had a normal intellectual capacity at follow-up.

In the United States, a sample of forty-eight children diagnosed with autism was followed up in late adolescence (McGovern & Sigman, 2005). Almost all persons were still diagnosed with an ASD, but their parents described improvements in the areas of social interaction, repetitive or stereotyped behaviors, adaptive behaviors, and emotional responsiveness in adolescence compared to middle childhood. The adults with autism who were able to live independently and hold jobs typically displayed good cognitive and communication skills despite their social deficits. Barnhill (2007) studied the course of Asperger's disorder into adulthood and found that those persons who achieved adaptive functioning levels continued to experience some impairment in employment, perception, social isolation, motor skills, and mood, with depression being a common condition.

Early diagnosis is important so that intervention can begin as soon as possible (Rogers & Vismara, 2008). Parental concern is a more important factor than pediatric testing in identifying a child with ASD (Mandell, Novak, & Zubritsky, 2005). Parents often voice concerns a year earlier than diagnosis formally takes place (Harrington et al., 2006). Researchers at the CDC found that children with ASD were initially evaluated at a mean age of forty-eight months, but were not diagnosed until sixty-one months (Wiggins & Cather, 2006). Other risk mechanisms for the course of autism include the child's aggression and self-injury behaviors, which compromise home and community place-ments (Gadow, DeVincent, & Schneider, 2008).

Standard Interventions

The Importance of a Comprehensive Focus

Comprehensive interventions for persons with ASD are defined as small-group or one-on-one behavioral and educational interventions that are delivered for at least ten to fifteen hours per week for a period ranging from months to years (Shattuck & Grosse, 2007). Unfortunately, no intervention has been shown to change the core features of ASD to an extent that the person is able to achieve normative levels of functioning. Still, steps may be taken to help the person make significant gains. The range of interventions should include special education, family support, behavioral management, and social skills training for persons with higher-functioning ASD. Medications may be used to control behavioral symptoms. Complementary and alternative medicines are also available that parents often find appealing (Harrington et al., 2006).

Applied behavior analysis (ABA) involves the examination of the antecedents of a problem behavior and its consequences. Any avoidable antecedents for a problem behavior are removed, and desirable behaviors are broken down into their component parts and introduced. Positive reinforcement is then provided after a child's desired behavior. ABA has been shown to facilitate improvements in adaptive, cognitive, and language skills, and to reduce problem behavior (Seida et al., 2009).

Rogers and Vismara (2008) concluded their systematic review with the following guidelines for effective autism early intervention programs:

- Treatment of unwanted behaviors should follow the principles of ABA.
- Building functional communication skills is a core aspect of effective treatment.
- Children need to be engaged in meaningful, age-appropriate learning activities that provide adaptive skills for use in multiple settings. Client choice should be used when possible.
- Effective early intervention can occur in a number of settings as long as there are coherent teaching plans administered at a high frequency throughout the day and across multiple settings, ongo-

ing monitoring of the child's progress, and the generalization of skills to natural settings.

- Peer interactions are critical in fostering the child's social growth.
- Ensuring the generalization of new skills is essential, so relevant adults and other children should be prepared to support them.
- Parents and family members need to be included in the intervention, in part to secure supports for themselves.

For adolescents, interventions should emphasize the acquisition of adaptive and vocational skills to prepare the individual for independent living. Sexual development in adolescence brings additional behavioral problems that may be addressed with sexual education and behavioral interventions (Holter, 2004). Because public school responsibility ends when a person reaches age twenty-two, the identification of community resources and support for adults in planning for long-term care is critical. Options include independent (or semi-independent) living, living with parents, foster homes, supervised group living, and institutions for those who need intensive, constant supervision (NIMH, 2007).

Medications

Drug intervention may help with aggression, self-injury, inattention, and stereotyped movements, and these improvements may help the person become more amenable to other interventions (des Portes, Hagerman, & Hendren, 2003). For the client's anxiety, selective serotonin reuptake inhibitor drugs may be helpful (Leskovec, Rowles, & Findlay, 2008). General attention in ASD children may be improved through the use of stimulants (Oswald & Sonenklar, 2007). Evidence for significant reductions in hyperactive symptoms is strongest for the antipsychotic drugs (particularly risperidone), psychostimulants, and naltrexone. Some evidence of the benefits of risperidone in irritability, repetition, and social withdrawal is apparent (Jesner, Aref-Adib, & Coren, 2007).

For reducing aggression, antipsychotic medications, including risperidone, olanzapine, and clozaril, may be effective. Naltrexone has been posited to block opioids that may be released during self-injurious repetitive behaviors. Biopterin (a naturally occurring enzyme) supplements appear to elicit small improvements in language and social functioning in some persons with ASD (Tager-Flusberg, Joseph, & Folstein, 2001).

Complementary and Alternative Interventions

The National Center for Complementary and Alternative Medicine groups these therapies into four domains: mind-body medicine, biologically based practices, manipulative and body-based practices, and energy medicine. The most commonly used of these interventions for ASD fall into the categories of biologically based and manipulative and body-based practices. Hanson and colleagues (2007) reported that 41 percent of respondents endorsed benefit with dietary and nutritional treatments, whereas Wong and Smith (2006) found that 75 percent of respondents believed that these treatments were helpful.

The following two examples highlight special challenges to recovery practice that are inherent in working with persons who experience ASD. In these examples, the social workers needed to engage in vigorous advocacy because their consumers experienced service inadequacy, required assistance in managing cross-state linkages, dealt with adverse effects of shifts in public policy, and appealed the denial of insurance coverage. The mixed outcomes of each illustration underscore the difficulty of upholding the recovery philosophy's commitment to creating social institutions that are more inclusive and accepting of persons with ASD. The first story is presented as a first-person narrative by Amy, a social worker and one of this chapter's coauthors.

The Young Adult

Michael was a twenty-one-year-old male with autistic disorder; he was diagnosed at the age of three. Prior to adolescence, Michael struggled with socialization and communication, but did not exhibit any harmful behaviors. At age sixteen, however, his parents noticed an increase in Michael's level of frustration when he was denied access to desired items. His resulting behavior led to episodes of property destruction and physical aggression. At nineteen, Michael was admitted to our residential treatment center because of a steady increase in this behavior. The center was located out of state; the state in which he resided did not offer any services for his level of need. Many programs there had denied services to Michael based on his diagnosis and symptoms, largely because he was aggressive toward adults and peers. After his assessment it was found that, on average, he engaged in five episodes of aggression per day, with 75 percent of those episodes causing harm to others (bruising, scratching, pinching, biting, hair pulling). He also displayed attention-seeking (to get a reaction from adults or peers) and escape (to avoid or delay performing a task) behaviors, including property destruction, loud vocalizations, running away from others, and noncompliance. Although many persons with autism struggle in these areas, Michael's adaptive behaviors included appropriate communication (he could request preferred items and activities) and the ability to independently attend to many activities of daily living (e.g., hygiene, leisure skills).

I served as Michael's primary behavior analyst. Our team developed an initial treatment plan to increase Michael's adaptive behaviors while targeting his inappropriate behaviors. The plan included medication management and ABA interventions that included providing minimal attention to problem behaviors followed by positive consequences for appropriate behaviors, positive reinforcement of alternative behaviors (behaviors that Michael engaged in instead of the problem behavior), social skills groups, and token economy systems. A primary intervention was that of functional communication training: 80 percent of problem behaviors exhibited by persons with autism are the result of communication frustrations. The other staff and I implemented mass communication trials daily so that Michael could practice appropriate requesting. Michael reponded well to these interventions, and within seven months he had met his goals and was ready for discharge to his home environment.

Our treatment team identified four primary services for Michael's aftercare: in-home ABA, medication management, social work services for the family, and special education services. It was my responsibility as the social worker to coordinate services with the ABA provider in Michael's hometown. I reviewed Michael's treatment plan, including the current behavior reduction and skill acquisition data, with a service provider at the new agency. Discharge planning between the treatment team, Michael's mother, and the new ABA provider included discussion about the preferred type of ABA and a description of our services. Because Michael had an extensive set of skills in his repertoire, we recommended a consultative model of aftercare so we could provide ongoing support to the new service providers. Fortunately, Michael's aftercare treatment plan fit with the service resources at the new facility to help ensure a successful transition: one-to-one staffing, functional communication training, positive reinforcement for appropriate behaviors, a token economy system, and planned ignoring (providing no attention to nonharmful, attention-seeking behaviors). Michael enjoyed listening to music, playing on the computer, working puzzles, reading books and magazines, and drawing, and having these skills in his repertoire made for a successful transition. Although Michael required twenty-four-hour supervision, he did not need constant monitoring. Two months after returning home, Michael was maintaining his skills and making further progress. Michael's parents were pleased with the transition.

So far, so good. Unfortunately, the service system soon failed Michael and his family. Within three months of his discharge, the state's Medicaid plan discontinued the coverage of ABA services for individuals over the age of eighteen. In addition, due to limitations in state funding, there were no ABA services available at Michael's school. Within six months of being home, then, Michael began deteriorating and our residential facility received a referral for Michael's readmission. The reasons for the referral included Michael's inadvertently drowning the family's dog in the swimming pool, as well as injuring his eighty-year-old great-aunt, punching holes in walls, and ripping doors off their hinges.

Michael was readmitted to our residential facility several months after his twentieth birthday. The presenting problems included aggression toward others, property destruction, and noncompliance. Due to these variables being consistent with his first admission, our treatment plan was similar to the earlier ones. A heavy emphasis in our program is on structure, following a schedule, reinforcement, and functional communication. Gradually, Michael's maladaptive behaviors decreased and he was again meeting criteria for discharge. As the treatment team began diligently searching for adult services that would meet Michael's needs, Michael was denied coverage by his insurance company, which stated that "he no longer meets criteria for a residential level of care." Our facility had one week to find a placement or in-home services for Michael, who was approaching twenty-one years of age.

Adult services for persons with moderate to severe autism are limited. Group homes exist, but in most states Medicaid does not cover the level of support required for an individual with autism. There is also a long waiting list for adult services. In the state where Michael resided, a person was only considered to be in crisis (and thus move to the top of the waiting list) if he or she was homeless, had no immediate family to provide care, or was in imminent danger to self or others. Michael did not meet any of those criteria. As a recovery-minded social worker, I wanted to secure housing for Michael in a supportive and relatively nonrestrictive place, but this was proving difficult.

On the day of Michael's denial, his parents appealed the insurance company's decision, with my support. During such an appeal, the insurance company is mandated to cover expenses for the person to remain at the current placement. A guardian-initiated appeal includes a documentation review by an administrative law judge followed by a hearing. Our program director was invited to testify and submit a letter for review, which I helped to compose and is excerpted below:

To Whom It May Concern:

We believe that Michael's progress is primarily attributable to 24-hour staffing support in a highly structured environment. Michael engages in low problem behaviors during high levels of engagement. He responds well to intense behavior programming. Michael requires assistance with many daily living activities. Although Michael no longer meets criteria for a psychiatric residential facility with 24-hour nursing and psychiatry, he does require 24-hour support. It is apparent that Michael would regress in a less supported environment as evidenced by his behavior during the six months after he returned home. Michael would continue to progress in a residential school setting that is able to provide 24-hour staffing support.

Based on the testimonies of his family and some professionals, and the available clinical information, the judge ruled that Michael should remain at our residential facility until aftercare services had been identified by the center and insurance company. Five months after the hearing, Michael remained at the residential placement—a highly restrictive, locked facility. He continued to display only low levels of problem behavior and did not meet criteria for this type of placement. Additional services have not been identified because there are no services that might adequately meet his needs. An ideal program (in-home or out-of-home placement) for Michael would include the following: behavior analytic programming; one-to-one staffing ratio; leisure, vocational, and daily living curricula; exposure to functionally appropriate peers to promote socialization; parental or caregiver support and training; medical services; and various other individualized supplemental services.

It is unfortunate, but Michael's example is becoming more and more the norm. With its increased prevalence, the number of adults with autism in the next few years will reach record high levels. Although there is an increase in awareness of this challenge, there is a startling lack of response regarding service development. Persons like Michael may be thought to have limited recovery potential, but they deserve the utmost respect of their communities by being able to share as much as possible in community life.

Amy continues her story with some thoughts about policy issues.

Recovery Obstacles During the Transition to Adulthood

At age twenty-two, persons with Individualized Education Programs (IEPs) age out of the public school system. This is the turning point where school services end and adult services should begin. Many states do not have adequate services for persons with autism, primarily due to restrictions in funding, education, training, and the lack of awareness of the need for adult intervention.

Advancing Futures for Adults with Autism (AFAA) is an advocacy organization designed to meet the recovery needs of adults with autism in society. Through autism congresses, national town meetings, and expert panels or think tanks, AFAA pursues its mission to resolve the following questions (www.afaa-us.org, 2011):

- How do we, as a society, help this group of citizens achieve their rightful place as participating members of society and in so doing transition from an all-too-common status as dependent, to engaged, involved and, ideally, tax-paying members of their communities? Among the pressing questions to be answered are these:
  - Where are we? (current state of the art in residential, vocational, recreational, transitional programming)
  - Where do we want to go? (new models of support that will allow individuals to have full and meaningful lives)
  - How will we get there? (Projects or initiatives, strategies, policy changes)

In November 2009, I was sent by my treatment center to participate in the AFAA National Town Hall Meeting. More than a thousand participants gathered in Chicago or in one of fifteen satellite locations. Participants included adults with autism, family members of adults with autism, community service providers, public officials, community members, and organization sponsors. The town hall was organized so that each of the round tables consisted of at least one member from each group listed above. The meeting agenda focused on crosscutting issues, including housing, employment, community life, and a five-year advocacy plan. The goals of the town hall meeting were to initiate discussion on the needs of adults with autism, develop needs assessments based on priorities, and begin the planning stages.

The recovery philosophy focuses on client empowerment, reducing social stigma, and collaborative treatment approaches. There has been very little research on the recovery model and autism, however, especially in cases where the peson is significantly impaired. During the town hall meeting, I had the opportunity to speak with two adults who have high-functioning autism about the challenges they encounter on a daily basis. Sonya is an eighteen-year-old female and Joe is a fifty-five-year-old male. Their views directly speak to the relevance of the recovery philosophy.

Each discussion area at the town hall meeting was divided into strategies. One strategy discussed was to "ensure that adults with autism have access to the supports they need to develop the life skills necessary to live safe, independent and productive lives." Both Sonya and Joe had strong opinions about this strategy. They both indicated that too often supports and life-skills training focuses on decreasing behavior that is not socially acceptable. They believe it is their right to engage in these behaviors regardless of their environment. For example, Sonya stated that if she were restricted from engaging in self-stimulatory behaviors, she would feel more stress and anxiety. She also challenges the basis of the question, "What is socially acceptable?" She often observes "typically developing individuals" engaging in bizarre behaviors, yet their behavior is not interrupted. Related to this point, Wehman, Smith, and Schall (2009) have stated that there are often challenges to maintaining the dignity of persons with autism. Many of the stereotypical behaviors in which these persons engage (e.g., spinning, rocking, rituals) may be embarrassing and cause demeaning reaction from onlookers, but they are harmless to others and possibly helpful to the person. It is thus a challenge to maintain dignity while promoting individuation. Joe felt very strongly about behavior plans written to decrease so-called problem behaviors without having input from the individual. Joe stated that, through his state's department of developmental disabilities, an individual is assigned a case manager and behavior analyst. He stressed that the consumer's involvement in the development of the plan should be the number one priority. He also stated that, too often, interventions are based on general research data rather than on the individual's perceptions or needs.

Another issue that prompted much discussion at the conference was related to employment: the need to increase and expand the number of successful programs that match adults with autism with meaningful jobs. Joe stated that individuals with autism are put into a limited set of employment categories: janitorial, housekeeping, food services, and landscaping. Job coach programs are created in these environments and persons with autism do not typically have access to other job opportunities. Joe stated that it is frustrating to be categorized as such rather than be matched with a job dependent on his skills, strengths, and interests. Fortunately, some states do have customized employment programs (Wehman et al., 2009).

The viewpoints of Sonya and Joe reflect key concepts of the recovery philosophy: empowerment, social stigma, and treatment collaboration. These consumers were adamant that they did not need to be fixed, but rather required assistance in managing their self-identified problem areas. There should be a greater balance between individual needs and services available.

Amy's Commentary

Michael, Joe, and Sonya reflect the range of levels of functioning in the autism spectrum. Recovery practice suggests that autism services for adults should be highly variable, given this broad spectrum, so that each person can achieve his or her highest level of recovery. The range of services (e.g., vocational, recreational or leisure, behavior management, residential) should be based on level of functioning (severely impaired to Asperger's disorder) rather than broad stereotypes. Skill workshops, job coaching, day treatment programs, and supported employment programs are just a few of the possible employment programs. Evidence-based practices, developed through research, should be adopted throughout adult services for persons with autism. Best practices now include ABA, reinforcement, picture schedules, communication systems, and provision of consequences that relate to the function of the behavior

(Cooper, Heron, & Heward, 2007). At the same time, services should be individualized.

In addition to the above, I attempted to remain true to recovery practice for Michael in my attention to the following:

- The values of empowerment, antistigma, and treatment collaboration with formal and informal providers. My goals were to help Michael earn his chance to live independently, be accepted in his environment despite his limitations, and give both him and his caregivers a strong voice in helping those goals come about.
- Envisioning a society that will accommodate persons like Michael, rather than assuming that interventions should focus on his needs to make certain (perhaps unrealistic or harmful) changes to cause him to fit in to the status quo.
- Advocacy, in my continuous efforts to secure the funding and service opportunities for Michael that would promote his functioning potential. Services for persons with autism are especially fragmented, which results in many consumers falling out of the service system. Much advocacy activity takes on a confrontational tone, because service providers are not always willing to look creatively beyond constraints in helping with a consumer's goals.

The Young Child

Daniel is a six-year-old boy diagnosed with autism and a rare neurotransmitter disease. Between the two disorders, Daniel has encountered serious natural and service-system obstacles to his physical and emotional development, and these will likely continue. His physical problems include delays in language and communication, delays in the development of gross and fine motor skills, and impaired social cognition. Daniel's struggles are made more bearable by an excellent support system comprising his family, friends, caretakers, and service providers. Despite these assets, service limitations prevent the young boy from functioning at his potential. Both social and agency advocacy activities are prominent in the recovery activities of his social worker.

When Daniel was an infant, his parents sensed he was not developing normally. His mother had done research on developmental milestones and knew what to expect of a typical child. Daniel was not meeting those milestones, and was exhibiting other behaviors that served as warning signs that he might not be "normal." These early indicators included uninterrupted sleeping through the night and a lack of self-preservation instincts such as protecting his head and neck. Daniel's parents shared these observations with their pediatrician who, after an examination, decided that Daniel should undergo additional testing by a hospital neurologist. It was eventually discovered that Daniel's urine levels had a spike in a neurotransmitter enzyme known as GHB. The accumulation of GHB in one's blood is a telltale sign of a debilitating disease known as Succinic Semialdehyde Dehydrogenase Deficiency. The formal diagnosis of this disease, which causes chronic neurological and cognitive defects, seizures, and impairments in language development, auditory perception, and motor coordination, was eventually confirmed. Daniel was just six months old.

Daniel's parents were almost bankrupted by paying for their son's medical services because there was no insurance coverage available for this rare disorder. At the age of two, however, Daniel was given the additional diagnosis of autism, when his perseverative behaviors began to manifest themselves. Ironically, this diagnosis proved to be beneficial to Daniel's well-being because it enabled him to qualify for government-supported services that he would need to improve his quality of life. Daniel's parents were able to obtain health-care funding that enabled them to stop paying out of pocket for some of Daniel's treatments and qualify for therapies he was not yet receiving. It was also at this time that Daniel's parents received a referral to a social worker who would help them navigate their way through the health service system.

Brittany is a social worker who, through her agency, provides case management services to persons with autism and their families. She understands the fragmented service system and knows how to help families advocate for government funding. She also maintains a recovery focus, which in this context means helping Daniel secure a lifestyle that is comfortable, accommodating, and facilitative of his ongoing development. In the four years since Daniel's autism diagnosis, he has participated, with Brittany's assistance, in many interventions, most of which have been at least partly successful. Still, Daniel's parents, with Brittany's advocacy support, have had to fight for many of these services and have spared no cost to ensure that Daniel can maximize the quality of his young life. These interventions are summarized next.

Daniel has been receiving physical therapy since six months of age when he was first diagnosed with the neurotransmitter disease. Daniel's physical therapist worked on skills including sitting up, rolling over onto his stomach and back, and crawling. Over time, his therapy has helped him develop gross motor skills such as balancing, strengthening core muscles, kneeling, scooting, pulling up, standing, and most recently, walking. Daniel's fine motor skills have also been honed during these treatments.

In addition to physical therapy, Daniel has been receiving speech therapy since age one. This treatment was especially hard for Daniel's parents to obtain. Daniel had just begun early intervention therapy but the regional medical board in charge of allocating services was not convinced that he required speech therapy. Daniel's parents were forced to advocate on behalf of their son at educational meetings. Many of these discussions became quite intense and so difficult to resolve that Daniel's parents had to enlist the help of an educational consultant in order to win their case. There is no doubt that speech therapy was and still is needed: Daniel lacks a reliable capacity to communicate. His speech skills categorize him as an emergent speaker. He is not yet able to choose the sounds he makes at all times. Daniel has seen many speech therapists over the years, some privately and others employed by the schools he has attended.

Daniel has also received both occupational and feeding therapies. During occupational therapy, he has been prompted and taught to develop his fine motor skills and to use both hands while engaging in activities. Feeding therapy was initiated after Daniel's doctor suspected that he was aspirating liquids (taking them into his airway) instead of swallowing them. When this was confirmed, Daniel underwent treatments to help him utilize the muscles in his mouth and throat to direct liquids where they needed to go. Daniel's parents must still feed Daniel finely processed foods that are soft in consistency. Daniel does not yet know how to chew food independently, and foods that are hard in consistency would represent a choking hazard.

It should be emphasized that Daniel's parents were organizing their lives around his care all this time, and spent hours each day engaging in the exercises their son needed to develop his skills. They were fully willing to act in this manner, but part of the role of the recovery social worker is to help families to obtain professional services so they can get some relief from their ongoing care responsibilities.

When Daniel received the secondary diagnosis of autism and his parents were able to obtain government assistance, he became eligible for ABA in his home, which was a major turning point in his development. Prior to utilizing this service, however, Daniel's parents had decided to enroll him at a specialized school that was geared toward young students with autism and developmental delays and that used ABA as its primary teaching method. Brittany helped to coordinate Daniel's treatment regimen there. It turned out that the school, although helpful for some persons with autism, did not fit Daniel's needs as well as his parents and social worker had wished. One of Daniel's unique characteristics, which is a great strength, is that unlike many people with autism he has become a social being. He enjoys interacting with adults as well as other children, and he is motivated to learn from other children through interaction and observation. The specialized school that Daniel attended did not have the social environment that would benefit Daniel. The work schedule at the school was also too rigid for Daniel, who was just two years old at this time. His attention span had not developed enough to tolerate long work sessions.

After one year, Daniel's parents decided to remove Daniel from the specialized school and, following consultation with Brittany, enrolled him at a local public school in an early intervention classroom. Brittany also linked them with another agency so they could hire an in-home ABA instructor who would meet with Daniel each day after school. This new educational arrangement worked well. Daniel was able to socialize with children of similar age and different backgrounds in an environment that was structured but that focused on his unique needs. Then, when he came home in the afternoon, Daniel received ABA instruction for his academic and behavioral needs. A modified schedule of this arrangement is still in place for Daniel today.

Commentary

Daniel is progressing slowly. With Brittany's monitoring, he continues to receive many health services but their frequency has tapered from the daily and weekly regimens he once experienced. Daniel's parents continue to pay out of pocket for some treatments, whether they be extra sessions or unfunded services. Daniel is likely to require intensive professional services for the rest of his life. This kind of consumer is, unfortunately, not highly valued by most members of our society and thus faces many limits in securing funded support services, which presents a frustrating state of affairs for his family.

In this context, Brittany's recovery activities with Daniel and his parents can be summarized as follows:

- She spent much of her work time engaging in advocacy activities with Daniel's parents, trying to obtain services by battling in boardrooms and then waiting interminable amounts of time to find out if service applications had been accepted.
- She maintained allegiance to fundamental values of recovery that might be overlooked by some practitioners in the context of Daniel's limitations (hope, family self-direction, individualized action, consumer and family empowerment, holism, nonlinearity, strengths-basis,

peer support, given his social skills), respect, and family responsibility.

- Despite the fact that Daniel is receiving services, it is possible that as he gets older he will continue to live in environments more restrictive than they might be if additional service options, based on a greater social resolve to accommodate the needs of such persons, were available. Brittany's recovery efforts will continue to focus on helping Daniel qualify for a normal lifestyle to the extent that his disabilities will allow.

Summary

Social workers are not qualified to intervene directly into medical aspects of intervention for persons who experience ASD, but they can provide the behavioral and systems interventions described in this chapter. In their case management roles, social workers can coordinate the interventions provided by a range of professionals and help consumers and their families plan for long-term professional involvement. As the social or recovery model of practice becomes more prominent, social workers will be able to apply their strengths perspective toward greater natural support system development, and their advocacy perspectives will help the larger community adapt to the needs of persons with ASD.

Major Chapter Learning Points

- Interventions for persons with ASD must be comprehensive to be effective, which demands that the recovery practitioner coordinate the activities of many professionals and support the implementation of the recovery philosophy among them as much as possible.
- Persons who experience ASD are often unable to advocate for themselves, so recovery practice is usually characterized by a high level of advocacy on the part of the practitioner.
- Much recovery practice with persons who have developmental disabilities is focused on changing environments to become more accommodating to them, rather than altering consumers' behaviors to better fit with existing social norms and supports.

- With ASD, a recovery orientation requires the practitioner to take a broad view of what is termed "acceptable" behavior.
- Recovery from the ASD is inevitably a slow process and requires a great deal of patience from the practitioner.

Questions for Reflection or Discussion

1. Review the major values of the recovery philosophy in chapter 2. Which of them might be operationalized differently when working with persons who have ASD?
2. To what extent should recovery practitioners advocate for a broader acceptance of symptomatic behavior of persons with severe ASD, when many of those behaviors are offensive to members of the general population?
3. What skills are required of a recovery practitioner who must engage in cross-system advocacy? How can these skills be acquired?
4. In an effort to help society become more accommodating to persons with severe ASD, what range of resources should be developed for both consumers and their caregivers?

Chapter 11

Endings in Recovery Practice

This chapter addresses the process of ending relationships in recovery practice. The importance of attending to the ending of an intervention is to ensure that both the social worker and the consumer achieve a sense of closure. That is, both parties should understand why the relationship is ending and process the experience of that ending together. The consumer should leave the relationship with a sense of self-empowerment and respect, a capacity for self-direction, the sense of having been supported, and, above all, hope that his or her recovery will continue. Closure may include the worker's and consumer's acknowledgment of feelings about the relationship, which may enhance their mutual confidence in developing positive relationships in the future, professional and otherwise. This chapter includes attention to the following eight ending guidelines for recovery-minded social workers to incorporate into their practices, along with examples of how they may unfold (Walsh, 2007):

- Deciding when to implement the ending phase
- Anticipating the consumer's and one's own reactions
- Appropriately spacing the remaining meetings
- Reviewing the relationship
- Reviewing and generalizing recovery gains
- Planning for ongoing recovery
- Setting conditions and limits on future contact
- Participating in ending rituals

The manner in which these tasks unfold will depend on circumstances of the ending, the influence of agency policies, and the personalities of the participants. They all represent mutual processes, although the emphasis here is on how the social worker can initiate them constructively.

Deciding When to Implement the Ending Phase

The social worker and consumer should know from the outset that their working relationship will end at some time. The social worker may be very clear about this ("We are authorized to meet five times") or address the issue in general terms ("We can work together as long as it takes for you to achieve your goals"). Some guidelines for the social worker's looking ahead to the ending phase of intervention include

- Explaining any anticipated time limits to the consumer during their first meetings;
- Raising the topic of ending criteria at regular intervals;
- Asking the consumer at the end of every meeting or session how he or she is experiencing the intervention (thus, providing each session with an ending phase); and
- Utilizing concrete measures of progress so that both parties can see the endpoint as it approaches, however near or far away

Some consumers indirectly indicate a desire to end a recovery relationship. They may express increased confidence and share more reports with the social worker of successes, satisfaction, and progress. Social workers usually base their decisions to end the relationship on various indicators of improved consumer functioning and goal attainment. Other criteria may include the consumer's stated wishes, environmental changes that mandate ending the intervention, and the increased availability of external support for the consumer. With family and group interventions, the social worker may notice members' increased mutual support and respect. "Negative" ending criteria include consumer dissatisfaction, the consumer's development of extreme dependence on the social worker, an absence of perceived consumer improvement, or restrictive agency policies. Still, because recovery is a nonlinear process, the practitioner should never assume that the absence of improvement over a period is a problem. Maintaining strict behavioral ending criteria may be counterproductive, because doing so elevates the social worker to the level of an authority figure. Furthermore, social workers need to distinguish between the consumer's readiness to end and their own desires to do so.

Social workers should not delay addressing relevant ending issues with consumers once they recognize the onset of the final phase. A reluctance to move forward in this way is unfortunately common and is often related to the social worker's ambivalence (Philip, 1994). Social workers rated as highly empathetic are at risk of spending too much time in the ending phase with consumers, while structured, task-focused social workers may move through the process too quickly (Holmes, 1997). The social worker is less likely to make errors in judgment if he or she incorporates the views of the consumer at these times.

When the social worker is leaving the agency and the consumer is staying, the practitioner must give thought to timing the announcement relative to the departure date. The social worker should make the announcement sooner rather than later, although specific decisions will depend on the nature of the relationship and program. The social worker should always share at least the basic facts of his or her departure, whether he or she is moving away, taking a new job, undergoing a career change, and so on, with the consumer.

In the first vignette, the social worker appropriately initiates an ending process but then has to return to a more intensive level of interaction with the consumer, only to have his later efforts at a planned ending disrupted by agency policies.

A Mobile Home Near the Woods

I am a social worker at Family Preservation Services, an agency that provides time-intensive in-home counseling and case management services. A regional Family Assessment and Prevention Team (FAPT), made up of public agency representatives, makes referrals to our agency for families that exhibit severe mental health and behavioral problems. Staff go to the consumers' homes three or four times per week, spending a great deal of time with all family members to help them learn to manage serious and long-term problems. An average visit is two or three hours, and the full intervention process can take six months or more.

I worked with the Anderson family for a full year. Mrs. Anderson (age thirty-eight and diagnosed with schizoaffective disorder), her live-in boyfriend (age thirty-five and unrelated to the children), two adolescent sons (ages sixteen and fourteen), and an adolescent daughter (age thirteen) had come to the attention of several legal and human service agencies because of their physical violence with one another. The mother had filed assault charges against each of her sons, but also had initiated fights with them at times, and with her daughter. They had recently moved from another state into a small, two-bedroom trailer in an isolated rural area. The family members were estranged from each other and disconnected from the nearby community. The FAPT team hoped that we could help them learn alternative ways of working out conflicts.

I was in the Anderson home quite a lot. The entire family was ambivalent about my visits, but this is typical of our consumers. Sometimes they were happy to see me, and other times I seemed to annoy them. In-home services are highly invasive, so in the best of circumstances families are relieved when we go away. But the Andersons made progress. Through my teaching, assistance with conflict mediation, role-playing, and modeling, they reduced their use of violence and increased their sense of contentment with one another. I connected well with Mrs. Anderson, who hoped that I could help her establish better control of the household. Even though the work was crisis oriented, I worked from a recovery perspective in helping her set goals of increased external support and self-direction, and I also helped her perceive how she could recognize and use her strengths to greater advantage. She—and, to a lesser extent, the other family members—became able to step back and think about their behaviors more carefully and to better control their impulses. After six months, I initiated a step-down ending process with the family, in which I gradually reduced my amount of contact with them to see if their positive changes would be lasting. I made clear to Mrs. Anderson, and she agreed, that she was making appropriate choices in setting limits on the behavior of her children. I moved from ten, to six, and then to three hours per week in their home. This process normally takes a few months. Unfortunately, the Anderson children's violent behaviors escalated as my time with them decreased. I was disappointed, but I was aware that recovery doesn't always proceed in a steady manner. I resumed seeing the family at nearly my previous level of intensity. While frustrated with the family dynamics, Mrs. Anderson expressed gratitude for my ongoing support.

After a year had gone by, FAPT decided that, despite the family's ongoing difficulties, the in-home program needed to end because of its expense. I disagreed with the decision, and my agency tried to work out a compromise with FAPT so that our intervention might continue with some regularity. In the end, this was not to be. My agency supervisor voiced an unfortunate reality of public social services—that if the family crashed later, they might qualify for other types of service. That is precisely what happened. One of the boys was soon removed from the home to a school for adolescents with emotional disabilities, and the girl was placed in foster care. After the termination of my services, Mrs. Anderson called me for assistance on a number of occasions, but I was not authorized to respond with personal contacts. I did make a special trip to their home (an unofficial visit that I did not get agency credit for) to review parenting strategies again with Mrs. Anderson. It was the last time I saw her. Mrs. Anderson was not happy, and wondered why she didn't get a say in the matter. I agreed with her, but needed to follow agency policy.

I understand the realities of public funding, but I felt disappointed with this outcome. I had no sense of closure with the family and was concerned that they were being left in a vulnerable position. My insistence that I couldn't visit them anymore was in violation of the recovery values of social worker–consumer equality and the process as being consumer driven. The abruptness of my ending with Mrs. Anderson made me wonder if she would be able to trust health-care professionals in the future. I attempted to process our termination for three weeks before I ended my visits with them, reviewing our work and helping them stay focused on their newer coping behaviors. But Mrs. Anderson seemed angry with me.

Anticipating the Consumer's and One's Own Reactions

In recovery practice, the social worker and consumer may develop an intense, emotionally charged relationship, and its ending may be a significant experience for both parties. In preparation for that event, the social worker should attend to the following:

- Consider factors that are likely to influence the consumer's response to ending. These include the degree of the consumer's positive change, satisfaction with the intervention, personality style, previous experiences with loss, and range of current supports. A consumer's attachment to an agency where he or she will receive ongoing services can help him or her better manage an ending with a social worker (Harrigan, Fauri, & Netting, 1998).
- Use supervision or peer feedback to assess his or her own levels of attachment to the consumer as the relationship ends. The worker can use this input to recognize more clearly his or her feelings about the course of the intervention. The social worker can also benefit from feedback about the possibility of his or her own avoidance or minimization of the significance of the process to the consumer.

The professional relationship represents only one portion of a consumer's activities of daily living, and the consumer's reaction to the ending is influenced by what else is happening in his or her life. Does the consumer have other people to rely on for positive interaction? Does he or she interact with others who are respectful and who promote self-direction? Can the consumer seek out help from others when needed? Is the consumer involved in other productive life activities? Is he or she optimistic about the immediate future? If so, the consumer's reactions to the end may not be remarkable. Is the consumer lonely? Does the consumer have little to do during the day? Are his or her primary relationships conflicted? Is the consumer discouraged about the immediate future? If so, the consumer's reactions to the ending may be mixed.

The social worker should encourage the consumer to talk when there is a perceived lack of response to the ending process, but at the same time respect the consumer's need to be in control of regulating intimacy and distance. The consumer may feel sadness, relief, loss, anger, guilt, inadequacy, and anxiety. When consumers have mixed feelings, the worker can frame the ending process as a positive step in the consumer's mastery of separation, which is a challenge for most people. The worker may also share some of his or her own reactions, such as an enhanced sense of competence, pride, or even sadness, which highlight reciprocity in the relationship. The social worker must be careful, however, not to arouse feelings of concern in the consumer.

Be on guard for acting-out behaviors in consumers who experience strong reactions that they cannot articulate. If a consumer makes an abrupt break from the worker, outreach efforts should be no more active than in other phases of the intervention. That is, the consumer should ultimately be in control of managing the process.

The following vignette illustrates how surprised one social worker was about the consumer's reactions to the ending of their work.

The Business Cards

While I enjoyed all of my consumers, Delores was special. She was my first consumer at the mental health clinic, which was staffed by graduate students in social work and psychology. As a person with schizophrenia, the fifty-four-year-old African American woman presented numerous challenges for me throughout our relationship—from assessing her needs and cognitive abilities, to tailoring interventions to address her problems with disturbing hallucinations and disrupted relationships.

My work with Delores was challenging due to the vagueness of her thoughts and feelings. She often communicated with facial expressions and gestures, assuming they were sufficient to get her points across. She also suffered from episodes where she would lose time, when the voices in her head overwhelmed her. Panic attacks were common to her, so we worked on deep breathing, progressive relaxation, and visualization exercises that proved beneficial. I also used some solution-focused techniques to help Delores identify her strengths and ways to mobilize herself into constructive action. Delores remained anxious and isolative, but her sense of self-control was greater after our sessions, and she was more hopeful of developing some lasting peer relationships at a local clubhouse.

Because her moods were unpredictable and her thought processes often unclear, I initiated our ending process three months before our last session, after which time I would be graduating from school. In each session I reviewed our work together and acknowledged Delores' achievements. She never acted surprised when I routinely reminded her of the date of our last meeting, but I was not convinced that she understood our relationship would in fact end. As the number of our remaining sessions shrank, I focused our conversations on a balance between what Delores had achieved and what she might achieve in the future. Exactly one month from our last meeting, I started off a session commenting on the amount of time we had left. Delores burst into tears and was unable to talk for most of the hour. Despite our weekly termination discussions, Delores said that she didn't truly think it would happen. I could only remind her that our relationship would end, as bad as she felt about the fact.

I wanted to do something special for our last meeting. As a memento of our time together I had a set of business cards made for Delores to carry in her purse and place around her house. On one side of the card were our names and the dates we'd worked together. On the other side was a list of Delores' strengths. I suggested that she read these cards from time to time. Not only did she seem to appreciate the cards then, but a week later I received a note from Delores including one of the cards and a message that she hoped I'd keep one, too. Of course, I did.

Appropriately Spacing the Remaining Meetings

Many social workers and consumers adjust the frequency of their meetings during the ending phase, often spacing them farther apart. For example, a social worker and consumer may meet only half as often as usual for some period of time, and then perhaps even less frequently, until they stop meeting completely. The social worker may encourage the consumer to take more control over the scheduling, frequency, and length of meetings so he or she can pull away at a comfortable pace. With a tapering of meeting frequency, the consumer can test how he or she will feel without the social worker's presence and support.

Reviewing the Relationship

A consumer may be pleased or sad, or both, that an intervention is ending. Regardless of the affective tone of the event, the social worker should always address the course of their relationship. Two topics for reflective discussion can help the social worker process this issue. The first is that everyone's life includes continual oscillations between togetherness and parting (Sanville, 1982). The practice relationship and its ending hopefully offer opportunities for the consumer to experience increasingly comfortable oscillations. The consumer's decisions in these areas will symbolize taking more control of his or her life.

The second topic includes a review of the consumer's methods of coping with separation. The social worker may identify with and affirm the consumer's emerging ability to tolerate mixed feelings in relationships (Werbart, 1997). During the intervention, the consumer may have learned to accept and express anger toward the social worker at times, recognizing that such feelings do not prohibit a gratifying relationship. In short, the relationshp review will help the consumer reflect on his or her capacity to successfully engage in mutually supportive relationships in the future.

A process evaluation of the relationship may consist of the following discussion questions, initiated by the social worker:

- How collaboratively did we work together? Was I respectful of your situation?
- To what extent did our relationship contribute to your sense of self-direction and empowerment?
- What aspects of our work together did you find the most helpful? The least helpful?
- What suggestions would you have for me as I work with consumers in the future?
- Do you feel like I understood your holistic goals? Problems? Needs?
- How well were we able to communicate?

The following vignette illustrates a problem for the social worker that occurred when she did not think to directly address her relationship with the consumer before the ending of their work.

Fried Chicken and Warts

I met Pete when I worked in a residential program at a mental health center. Pete was in his fifties and lived in a government-subsidized apartment near the center. My job was to be a support for him: take him to the store and to the doctor, help with his household duties, link him to community services, and monitor his symptoms of schizophrenia. I wanted to help him learn to navigate independently through the community. We spent a lot of time together and had an easy rapport. He gave me, among other things, the secret to good fried chicken (cook it until all the blood comes out), and a remedy for getting rid of warts (rub them with a dirty dish towel, then bury that towel under the back steps). In addition to my practical functions, I provided Pete with companionship. He frequently told me stories of his mental illness, as if he were trying to make sense of what had happened to him. He also said he wanted to make a contribution to the world, although he couldn't articulate how.

Pete believed the medications helped him, but not because he had a mental illness. He said it made the demons that plagued him become quieter. Many of our talks started with a status report about his demons. Pete always struggled with the demons, except for the few times he excitedly told me that God had "taken them out of" him. He described the physical sensations that occurred as they were removed. Unfortunately, they always came back, and Pete would wonder what he had done to cause God to keep him in this condition.

Pete and I worked together for a year and a half and saw each other at least twice a week until I took a job at an inpatient psychiatric unit. When I said good-bye to Pete, I was sad at how accustomed he had become to professionals coming into and leaving his life. It seemed harder for me to say good-bye than it was for him. I kept up with him through a friend who worked at the center until she, too, left for another job. I always worried that Pete's case managers were not giving the same attention to his recovery that I had.

One day I was on the hospital unit when Pete was brought in on an involuntary detainment order. He was disheveled and yelling, and I noticed that his dentures were gone. I had never seen him angry with anyone besides his demons. Immediately I got on the phone with his residential counselor and demanded to know how he could get to this point before anyone noticed.

I felt sad and disappointed in the system. I felt even worse when I learned he had recently lost his apartment.

Pete was later discharged to a group home and then moved to North Carolina to be with his daughter. He called me one day while he was at the hospital to say he was back in a state facility. The last time I heard from him was on a Christmas Eve. He called to thank me for a carton of cigarettes I had sent him for the holiday. I had sent them against my better judgment when I remembered how he used to complain about the smoking restrictions in hospitals. I could have stayed in touch with Pete after that last phone call, but keeping the relationship going meant having to think about where he had started and where he was now. I didn't make a conscious decision not to call him again, but I never did. I'm not sure it was the right thing to do, just as I'm not sure I handled the ending with him in the best way.

I learned a lot from the experience. I learned that the more you care about consumers, the harder it is to see them move on, especially to lesser circumstances. I learned that ending is harder when you maintain some contact with the consumers but have no control over the care they get. I made the ending harder for myself by believing that no one else could care for Pete as well as me. I suppose it was naïve of me to believe that his stability over two years was mostly because of my work with him.

Part of what I carried away from my experience with Pete is that endings usually include ambivalence on both sides. Thinking about the relationship gets confusing when you commit your heart to the process. But I have come to believe that a certain amount of pain when someone is hurt or leaves is worth learning the secrets of great fried chicken and the cure for warts.

Reviewing and Generalizing Recovery Gains

Part of the process of achieving closure in the social worker–consumer relationship is looking back over the intervention and considering how the consumer has progressed in his or her recovery. This may include a formal evaluation, but more important includes helping the consumer informally review the worthwhile aspects of the intervention. The ending is an opportunity to put the pieces back together so the consumer can get a holistic picture of the process, and determine to what extent he or she can recognize an increased capacity for self-direction, individualized action, strengths, and peer support. The social worker may facilitate this task by

- Reviewing past intervention plans and the consumer's ultimate goals as a frame of reference for what has transpired;
- Sharing his or her own perceptions and memories of the process, focusing on key issues that indicated positive changes;
- Asking the consumer questions to stimulate his or her own reflections on the recovery process;
- Encouraging the consumer to ask significant others about any changes they have observed since the beginning;
- Inviting the consumer to write a journal summarizing his or her intervention experiences that the worker and consumer can review together; and
- In the case of families or groups, asking members to review with each other particular moments that indicated positive changes.

In some instances, the consumer may not perceive that he or she has made progress in recovery, and there may be unfinished business. Even so, it is important to help the consumer feel positive about the future when preparing to move on. Recovery, it must be reemphasized, is not a linear process.

What the consumer gains should be generalizable to other current and future situations. Part of the ending process thus involves the social worker and consumer reviewing how new knowledge and skills might be utilized in a variety of life situations. The social worker can facilitate this discussion with the following types of questions (DeJong & Berg, 2008):

- Let's step back and think about what you've accomplished here. How will you be able to use this in your life?
- You've reviewed with me today what you have achieved in our work together. Let me add some of my own observations about your recovery that go beyond what you've said. Let me know if they make sense to you.

- What have you learned about yourself that you can take with you to maintain your self-direction?
- Make a list of skills you have learned during our work together. Include on that list places where you might be able to use these new skills.
- Now that we are finishing, can you think of other challenges that you might be able to manage as a result of this experience?

A consumer's confidence can only be bolstered by the realization that he or she is now equipped to manage more issues than those for which he or she initially sought assistance. Recall, too, from chapter 4, that a variety of formal instruments have been developed for evaluating recovery-focused interventions.

Planning for Ongoing Recovery

The social worker and consumer typically devote much time during their final sessions looking ahead to the consumer's life after intervention with regard to managing recovery challenges. They anticipate what challenges the consumer is likely to face and how what he or she has learned can be retained. This process includes an acknowledgement of linkages to formal and informal support mechanisms that will contribute to the provision of ongoing support. The worker can help the consumer plan for these challenges with the following types of questions (DeJong & Berg, 2008):

- How might the challenge be manifested?
- Where might it occur?
- How frequently may it occur?
- What other persons and systems may be involved?
- What coping skills will you need to manage the challenge?
- What normal stress can you anticipate related to your life transitions?
- What resources will you need?
- What natural systems can you mobilize to manage your challenges?
- What obstacles might you experience while addressing your ongoing needs?

Another reflective topic for the ending process is a life review, which can help the consumer solidify a sense of identity: the social worker and consumer review where the consumer has been, his or her current status and new capabilities, and further recovery strategies the consumer may implement.

While the topic of ending rituals is discussed in depth later in this chapter, the following vignette shows how structured group activities can be effectively incorporated into endings to help consumers organize their thinking about ongoing recovery.

The Art Therapy Group

There are several ending activities that I use in my art therapy work at a short-term, inpatient substance abuse treatment facility. The average stay in the setting is about seven days, just enough time for consumers to become medically stabilized. My art therapy groups focus on the three goals of emotional expression, interpersonal connection (consumer to consumer, staff to consumer, and consumer to outside resources), and beginning-level behavioral change such as relapse prevention and coping responses based on understanding environmental cues. I try to generate several sources of support for consumers, utilizing community supports to broaden their repertoire of helping relationships.

A challenge in this setting is managing a consumer's sense of loss that comes with becoming intimate, even in a short amount of time, with the group, and then leaving, often abruptly. The consumers who remain also experience a sense of loss. One ending ritual that supports the consumer's appreciation of the power of community involvement is our good-bye ceremony. The consumer who is leaving sits in the middle of the group and each member reflects on his or her relationship with that consumer. Afterwards, the consumer communicates his or her feelings back to the group. This is a constructive process: members always emphasize strengths and remind the departing consumer of challenges he or she may face as a recovering substance abuser. This activity is affirming for the departing consumer as well as for those who remain, as they witness over and over again the significance of the community in supporting each one's recovery process.

One of my favorite activities that activates consumers' emotions related to loss and transition involves their artistic illustration of what they need to leave at the treatment facility and what they need to take with them. Examples of things to be left behind include panic, isolation, chaos, anger, fear, sadness, emptiness, negativity, betrayal, and resentments. Things to be cultivated from their experience often include serenity, happiness, gratitude, hope, a sense of self-direction, a positive attitude, support, and courage. One young male consumer, when asked to complete this activity, chose themes of chaos and serenity. He used a blue marker in his picture to symbolize both of these concepts, with a similar line quality to represent the seemingly disparate feeling states. Serenity was illustrated as a smooth, clear line, untangled from the web of chaos drawn on the paper's opposite side. Our group discussion focused on the parallels that exist between the two ideas, proposing that serenity can, in fact, be found in and arise out of chaos. We continued to dialogue about the line organization within the picture. It suggested the consumer's awareness of his own responsibility for emotional transformation and the existence of hope in the midst of addiction chaos. The group decided that active, personal responsibility coupled with a developing sense of faith in the recovery process would contribute to the chaos–serenity transformation visually represented in the consumer's artwork.

Another directed arts activity that helps consumers identify needed changes and promote supportive social networking is the recovery-related gift exchange. Consumers are paired and asked to create a recovery-related gift for their partners, based on what they think the partner needs. Consumers are asked to remain present focused. Examples of drawn gifts include candles that represent spirituality and wisdom, groups of family and friends that represent support and community connection, toolboxes that represent learned coping strategies, and clocks that represent a slowing down and increased mindfulness of purposeful daily activity. One consumer created a three-dimensional oyster with a pearl of wisdom inside, sharing with his partner his need to look inside himself for the power and strength to guide his recovery. Consumers often find humor and comfort in such interpersonal exchanges, benefiting from the giving of oneself and the ability to accept the gifts of others.

Setting Conditions and Limits on Future Contact

In recovery practice, the relationship between the social worker and consumer may be long term and include a great deal of informality because the social worker strives to avoid a hierarchical relaionship and empower the consumer to have input into the nature of their interactions. Still, once the social worker and consumer have their final session, they should understand how, when, and under what conditions they may initiate additional contact. The social worker may offer no options about future contact, or may informally invite the consumer to call if problems recur. The consumer's anxiety about ending may be diminished with the knowledge that he or she might see the social worker again.

The following vignette illustrates potential complications that may ensue when the issue of future contact is not addressed.

The Consumer Who Wouldn't Go Away

The domestic violence program where I worked offers counseling to women who are in abusive relationships. Often the women are living with their abusers. We try to help them learn new ways to cope with the domestic situation, provide them with information about community support resources, educate them about the cycle of violence, and in general help them take better care of themselves. We typically see consumers weekly for an hour. I worked with Sofia for three months and had a very difficult experience ending with her.

Sofia was in her early thirties, and in addition to her situation of domestic violence was diagnosed with bipolar disorder. She was not reliable about keeping our appointments, but I was never upset about this. She was living with an abusive husband who monitored everything she did. He often followed her to appointments with me and waited for her outside. He listened in on her phone conversations at their house. Sofia had two young children she was concerned about. I'd say that she came in for seven out of the twelve scheduled meetings. At those times, I helped her consider her existing social supports and tried to help her generate a sense of power to make changes in her life, as risky as they might be. When she missed a session, I'd call Sofia on her cell phone to see how she was doing and reschedule a meeting. I think she benefited from her counseling with me. She learned how to protect herself and her children.

I was scheduled to leave the agency on a particular date because my internship was ending, and Sofia knew this. I told her of my plans when we first met. She did not, however, show up for either of our last two scheduled appointments. I felt very unsettled about this. She had never missed two meetings in a row before. I wondered if this was a coincidence or Sofia's reluctance to say good-bye. I left without knowing the answer. I also felt bad that I did not know how she was getting along.

But that was not the end! Two months later Sofia called me at my home. She said that she and her husband were divorcing, and I should expect a subpoena to her child custody hearing. In one way it was good to hear from Sofia, but I was mostly upset about her call, and felt violated. We had never discussed the issue of ongoing contact, which in fact was discouraged by my agency. She had gotten my number out of the phone book. During the next month as the court case approached Sofia called me three or four more times at home. She was afraid for her safety, and felt that she didn't have any other support. I had mixed feelings about all of this. I didn't want to reject Sofia during her crisis, but I couldn't assume any official responsibility for her care. I kept asking her to call the YWCA or a local shelter for abused women. She always said she would, but she never did. This was a dangerous situation for me, for liability reasons and because her husband might see me as Sofia's collaborator. My mistake was not to be firmer with Sofia that she needed to seek professional assistance from people who could more realistically help her, and to stop calling me.

The court date came, and I was present but was not called to testify. I saw Sofia there, and we talked briefly. She certainly had appreciated my support. A few weeks later she called me again for some help, but this time I was firm about her need to contact other agencies for assistance. She said she would do so.

This was a stressful experience for me. In retrospect, I should have been clear during Sofia's first phone call that I could not have any more contact with her. I crossed boundaries in that posttermination period in ways that were risky. Still, I would have felt ambivalent about setting clearer boundaries because of ethical conflict I experienced with the agency, given my recovery orientation.

Participating in Ending Rituals

A ritual is any formal activity that is appropriate to a special occasion (Gutheil, 1993). It endows certain events with a sense of being special, and is most effectively observed during a time of change. Rituals symbolize continuity, stability, and the significance of personal bonds while helping people accept change and the need to move forward. Their structure provides a safe framework for participants to express feelings. During endings shared by social workers and consumers, rituals can affirm the importance of closure by bringing a special structure to their final interactions. While the social worker should always give the consumer the opportunity to take the initiative in designing such activities, several types of ending rituals are described below that social workers might use with recovering consumers.

Expressive tasks promote communication through art forms such as paintings, drawings, cutouts, music, poems, and stories; some of these were elaborated in "The Art Therapy Group" section above. These tasks tend to lower anxiety, move the participants past inclinations toward intellectualization, and stimulate emotional processing (Dallin, 1986). Themes on which the social worker might focus an activity include "good-bye to the old and hello to the new," "best and worst memories," what the consumer will miss the most and least about the sessions, how each person is experiencing the transition, and expectations about what lies ahead. The social worker's participation in the activity creates a parallel process, allowing him or her to experience feelings about the ending more fully.

A related strategy for consumers in transition is the worker's incorporation of status elevation ceremonies into social activities (Rouse, 1996). Endings that involve discharge from a psychiatric hospital or residential facility, for example, can be understood as transitional challenges, and to be times in which the consumer's relationships and sense of competence are in flux. The social worker can help the consumer manage transitions by empathizing with his or her loss of old attachments and helping the consumer develop new ones. Attending to this theme is consistent with the recovery philosophy's value of helping consumers to develop a sense of being normal in their social worlds.

The final vignette illustrates the power of simple rituals in the ending process. It also serves to summarize many basic tenets of the recovery process.

From the Laundromat to the Park

I once supervised a social work student named Jane who devised a marvelous and creative ending plan with a consumer. It provides an example of how the end of the professional relationship can be organized as a transition for the recovering consumer, moving on from temporary formal supports to permanent natural supports.

Our agency was a private multiservice community center, located in an urban neighborhood in a large city. It provided programs and resources to help consumers meet basic needs for food, shelter, and safety. A consumer in our job training program complained to me one day about one of her neighbors. She said the woman stayed in her apartment all day long with a screaming infant. This consumer was concerned about possible child abuse or neglect. I asked Jane to investigate the situation with a home visit. This is how Jackie became involved with our agency.

Jackie was a twenty-eight-year-old African American single mother of a two-month-old son. She had worked as a maid for a wealthy family until she became pregnant. Her boyfriend, the father of her child, had abandoned her, and Jackie had been fired from her job. Jackie had little money and was socially isolated and severely depressed. She was living on welfare benefits with nowhere to go and no one to turn to. Jackie was not abusing or neglecting her son, but she had many basic needs that were not being met. She was pleased to welcome Jane into her life, partly because the two women had so much in common. Jane was also African American, just a few years older than Jackie, and they shared similar backgrounds. Jane and Jackie became quite attached to each other. It was a testament to Jane's maturity as a practitioner that she realized the possible danger of her level of attachment to the consumer. She didn't want to become her consumer's friend, and she knew that Jackie might become too dependent on her. Jane wanted the consumer to develop the capacity for independent action. She understood that she needed to help Jackie achieve greater life stability and then end their relationship.

Jane and Jackie worked together for two months, spending many hours together each week. Jane helped Jackie acquire money and other benefits to live on, but she focused primarily on her social isolation. Jane wanted to help Jackie develop supportive friendships and she devised several creative strategies for bringing this about. First, all their early meetings took place at a neighborhood laundromat. This was the place where mothers with young children from the community were most likely to gather. Jackie met many other women there with similar interests and life situations, and these women became her friends. After a while, Jane targeted the neighborhood park as the site for their meetings. This was the second-most-popular gathering place for mothers with young children. The plan worked beautifully. Jackie's social isolation disappeared, and her mood gradually lifted.

Soon, Jackie was functioning well as a member of her community. She was confident in her ability to manage herself, had hopes for ongoing improvement, and felt good about herself, her friends, and her ability to support herself and her young son. It was time to end the intervention. Jane wanted their ending to be a celebration of Jackie's progress. The two women organized a big picnic in the park for their last meeting. Jackie invited her new friends and their children. All six of the women who came brought food and party items. They put a lot of preparation into the event because they knew that it was special for Jackie, to recognize how far she had come. It was ironic that Jane, the practitioner, was the only member of the group who would be leaving the group. It was a joyful occasion for all the women. Jane felt sad but very proud. Before she left the park that day, Jane took Jackie aside for a few minutes to reflect on their work and their relationship, and to affirm her progress. They hugged, and Jane drove off. Jackie stayed behind to help the other women clean up.

Summary

The manner in which the social worker–consumer relationship ends is important toward the goal of encouraging the consumer's investment in constructive future activities that will promote ongoing recovery. The purpose of this chapter has been to outline a set of common tasks for the social worker to address when the recovery relationship is coming to a close so both parties have the opportunity to process it in a positive way before going their separate ways. When the intervention has gone well, the consumer will function better and experience greater hope, self-direction, peer support, a capacity for individual action, a sense of empowerment, an awareness of his or her strengths, and greater self-respect. All of these outcomes reflect the basic values of the recovery philosophy. If the social worker has contributed to the advancement of any of these outcomes, he or she can feel pride in the work done.

Major Chapter Learning Points

- Attending to the ending of a recovery intervention is important for ensuring that both the social worker and consumer achieve a sense of closure—that is, an understanding of why the relationship is ending and an opportunity to process the experience.
- Closure may include the worker's and consumer's sharing of feelings about their relationship, which may enhance their mutual confidence in developing positive future relationships.

- Ending tasks for recovery-minded social workers may include deciding when to implement the ending phase, anticipating each party's reactions, appropriately spacing the remaining meetings, reviewing the relationship, reviewing and generalizing recovery gains, planning for recovery maintenance, setting conditions and limits on future contact, and engaging in transitional rituals.

Questions for Reflection or Discussion

1. Are there circumstances in which ongoing contact with a consumer who has ended his or her official work with a social worker would be appropriate? If so, what are they?
2. Were the social worker's posttermination actions in the "Fried Chicken and Warts" vignette appropriate? Why or why not?
3. What transitional rituals have you utilized in your own practice, and what others might you consider?
4. In the "A Mobile Home Near the Woods" vignette, how might the social worker advocate for policy changes that would allow social workers to have more discretion in their level and duration of service delivery?

Chapter 12

The Future of Recovery

The recovery movement, as an identifiable shift in thinking about the nature and course of mental illness, has been notable in the professional literature and service community for the past twenty years or so. The purpose of this final chapter is to summarize the state and future of the recovery philosophy from the perspectives of consumers, the mental health professions in general, and the social work profession in particular.

Generally speaking, it is difficult to speculate how the recovery philosophy will evolve in the coming years because it is such a broad concept. There are two contexts in which the perspective has evolved, each of which has different implications for the future (Davidson, O'Connell, et al., 2005). As a consumer movement, the term "recovery" refers to overcoming the effects of having a mental disorder in order to retain or resume a degree of control over one's life, and reclaiming one's sense of self and purpose. This perspective implies an emphasis on the consumer's self-directed recovery and a differential reliance on professionals. In this sense, practitioners embrace a recovery framework whenever they assist a person in realizing his or her potential as a unique human being who is not defined by an illness (Frese & Davis, 1997). Some consumers, of course, such as those participating in The Icarus Project (described in chapter 9), may reject the label of mental illness entirely. From the perspective of many professionals—that is, those who subscribe to a medical model bias—recovery refers to the amelioration of symptoms and other deficits associated with having a mental disorder, and assumes the importance of a strong ongoing role for professionals. One tension between the consumer and professional perspectives is the degree of leadership that is deemed appropriate for either group in the process.

The recovery philosophy calls for a service environment in which consumers have primary or collaborative control over decisions made about their own care. The values of the recovery philosophy are likely to persist indefinitely, with its present terminology or some other that might emerge. (What is "new" may become commonplace.) Research about the potentials of people with mental illnesses has validated the outcome and process perspectives on recovery, as well as the values of consumer empowerment and self-direction, and that will not change. What has made recovery unique is consumers becoming self-advocates and professionals becoming more sensitive to, and willing to invest in, the nonclinical aspects of consumer life. What is less certain than ongoing consumer organization, self-help, peer support, and advocacy is the future of the professional community's response to the recovery movement, and whether it will cooperate with consumers to an extent that requires changing some of its traditional roles (Ramon et al., 2009). Most fundamentally, professional strategies to promote recovery will need to focus simultaneously on the person and on his or her environment. What still needs to be expanded is professional appreciation for the holistic nature of recovery; it is likely that the various mental health professions will have a differential response to this challenge to expand based on their codes of ethics and preferred practice perspectives.

In considering the future of recovery, it is worth reviewing some of the related controversies within the mental health professions that were outlined in chapter 2.

Revisiting the Recovery Controversies

A focus on recovery may add to the burden of already stretched providers. Much recovery-oriented professional care is neither reimbursable nor evidence-based.   There is little evidence that recovery practice adds to the workload of service providers (Amering & Schmolke, 2009). In fact, one positive effect of the recovery movement is its encouragement of creative thinking about service delivery on the part of both consumers and professionals. Many recovering consumers are developing their own support services, which if anything might reduce their overall reliance on mental health professionals because of their demonstrated impact on quality of life (Nelson, Ochocka, Janzen, & Trainor, 2006). Furthermore, many agencies and professionals are developing recovery-oriented models of care, some of which have been described in this book, and are testing them for effectiveness. Several researchers (e.g., Torrey, Rapp, Van Tosh, McNabb, & Ralph, 2005) have generated principles for developing such practices, all of which include utilizing the insights of people who have experienced mental illness. It is likely that more of these services will demonstrate positive outcomes and become part of standard, reimbursable care.

Recovery can happen only after, and as a result of, professional intervention. This criticism gives prominence to the outcome versus process definition of recovery. Even so, the literature on long-term outcomes of mental illness has persuasively demonstrated that many persons can improve, whether or not they receive professional intervention. Furthermore, the literature, including the stories of survivors, demonstrates that there are indeed many paths to recovery, some of which involve much professional intervention and others that rely less on those resources. It emphasizes, too, that consumers can recover in some areas of life but not necessarily others, such as the physical, intellectual, emotional, relational, interpersonal realms, not all of which are associated with symptom reduction. Furthermore, as described in chapter 4, desired consumer outcomes are not necessarily the same as typical professionally generated outcomes. This criticism of recovery is likely to diminish in the face of further evidence that emerges regarding the recovery potential of all consumers.

Recovery-oriented care devalues the role of professional intervention. It has been shown throughout this book that there is a range of means by which consumers can address their recovery from mental illness, and some of these do not prioritize professional interventions. This does not devalue the roles of professionals, but relegates them to certain, but not all, aspects of consumer life. For most consumers, the mental health professions continue to be seen as critical resources for recovery, even as other peer-operated resources become available. Furthermore, because just over half the United States population with a mental illness receives services (58.7 percent of adults and 50.6 percent of children) (NIMH, 2012), it is possible that, if more consumers become aware through their recovery networks of available service options, the influence of professionals will be as great or greater than they are now. What is more problematic, and less certain as a future development, is whether the mental health professions will embrace the recovery value of egalitarianism in social worker–consumer relationships, and whether they will be willing to accept consumer practitioners. These new relationships might make those practitioners feel less professional or lower in status, compared to others who maintain society's medical perspective (Marshall et al., 2009).

Consumer choice increases providers' exposure to liability.   This concern, more than the others, has merit. Under current professional licensing laws it is possible that, as professionals promote consumer choice in service delivery, they could face liability risks when those choices have adverse consequences for the consumer (Warner, 2009). As one example, physicians are often not willing to provide consumer choice in medication evaluations (Deegan & Drake, 2006). In the words of one state mental health administrator, "Everyone supports recovery until something goes wrong." Research support for the benefit of increased consumer choice and consumer participation in service delivery will be required to adjust thinking on this point. Many professionals are not comfortable with providing broad choices, and many agencies have programs in place that are so structured as to not offer much if any choice to participants. If consumers are not satisfied with the choices available to them in a certain agency, practitioners should at least be prepared to make referrals to other resources and services.

Support for consumerism may represent an off-loading of responsibility from service providers.   A common concern of mental health professionals, certainly in public agencies, is the overwhelming demands of their jobs (Skovholt, 2001). Paperwork responsibilities are considerable, and caseloads are often high, so not all consumers receive as much attention as they may deserve. In these circumstances, practitioners may at times feel relieved when they lose consumers to dropouts. Still, these situations do not imply that practitioners want to avoid responsibility for their consumers, and most would be concerned about liability and ethical issues if they were to drop consumers who were not fully invested in agency-based interventions. To the extent that recovering consumers, when given choices, might opt out of certain aspects of professional treatment, this does not represent an off-loading of professional responsibility, but rather an openness to the availability of other sources of support for clients. On the other hand, if practitioners do take advantage of opportunities to do less with recovering consumers, without coordinating the range of service activities, they are clearly in violation of their ethical codes.

The language of consumerism may be used as a rhetorical device to reinforce the position of professionals.   This is a legitimate criticism—not of the consumer movement, but of the professions who may have a perspective on recovery that is more reflective of the medical model and its current power structure. Some would argue that even as the federal and state departments support the concept of recovery, they are doing so in word only, by not funding programs or providing other impetus for its development (Mechanic, 2008). That is, they may use the language to legitimize what they are doing, or want to do, without actually producing concrete changes.

Professional power may be exercised by limiting the range of decisions consumers can make and by shaping their roles to create the acceptance of expert authority.   Public service providers are realistically limited in providing consumer participation in the range of decisions they can make about the services offered them. Every agency-based professional is bound by the dictates of agency policies, program stipulations, licensing laws, and insurance company mandates, so that even if such a person has a consumer focus, he or she may not have the capability to realistically offer broad decision-making power to consumers. While this may be unfortunate, it is appropriate for each professional who is like-minded to do his or her best to offer decision making in the context of the services that may be available. This is not the same as protecting one's domain of expert authority, but it has similar consequences.

The recovery philosophy might unfairly assume that all consumers can fully recover from mental illness, and thereby stigmatize those who do not. This concern reflects another example of recovery being conceptualized as an outcome rather than a process. A careful reading of the recovery literature shows limited support for the notion of full recovery for most consumers, in the sense of their having no symptoms of mental illness. Recovery assumes that every consumer has the potential to engage in a unique process of recovery, and it makes no difference how and to what extent that unfolds. A stigmatization of consumers who are less able to achieve particular goals would represent a bastardization of the concept.

The recovery philosophy fails to recognize the difficulty of consumer empowerment. The capacity of the mental health professions to further the interests of consumers through empowerment has been a topic of concern among academic scholars, and there are at least two ways in which this is problematic (Barrett et al., 2010). Professionals may disapprove of, and thus negatively influence, what they perceive to be activities by some consumers that may put them at risk of failing, poor functioning, or backsliding. One of the major tensions between consumers and professionals is the role of professionals in assuming power in service decision making. Second, professionals may not be able to empower their consumers unless they themselves have more power among their peers in the service professions. For example, in interprofessional practice, one profession's recovery philosophy might not be endorsed by the others, and thus the consumer's activities may not be fully supported. This is likely to be an ongoing challenge as the meaning and scope of the concept of "empowerment" continues to be addressed and tested.

Social Work and Recovery

Despite the reservations noted above, it is likely that recovery will continue to be embraced by the social work profession. Social work values highlight a concern for the empowerment of oppressed people, support of each person's self-determination, and the person-in-environment perspective. Since a key point of the recovery philosophy is that it is not the role of practitioners to make all decisions for consumers, the basic values of recovery are consistent with those of the social work profession.

Among social work's most significant contribution to recovery has been its use of the strengths perspective in developing models of intervention (Rapp & Goscha, 2008). Through this perspective, consumer hope is nurtured both internally, by the perception that a person has strengths and resources necessary to reach his or her goals, and externally, by the cultivation of supportive relationships. The recovery process is dependent on consumers having options and choices, and social work values endorse offering choices and empowering consumers to the extent possible. One way this can be implemented is by providing consumers with information about treatment options and how they can experience personal growth. Critical consciousness of society's response to mental illness is also an important part of the social work value system. For example, although it uses the DSM and its language, the profession has always been open to considering alternatives, such as the person-in-environment system, which focuses a practitioner's attention on the four areas of a person's social, environmental, mental health, and physical functioning, and includes a strengths-based measure of coping (Karls & Wandrei, 1994; O'Neill, 2004).

Social workers must understand and accept that helping consumers make their own choices will ultimately be in the best interests of their recovery, even if the social worker believes that some actions may have adverse consequences. The recovery philosophy calls for social workers to support consumers' decisions to the best of their abilities. What remains to be seen is the extent to which social workers can partner with consumers whose capacities for good judgment (in the eyes of those professionals) seem at times to be impaired.

A challenge for social work is dealing with the reality that the public mental health system carries the assumption that psychiatric disorders are always and only organic, biological diseases. The Western social system endorses this idea as well, as evidenced by its holding the medical sciences in such high esteem. Social work will need to be active in the policy-making arena to promote consumer involvement in all levels of the service system, which is happening in many states. Still, recovery is unlikely to happen in the service system alone, and its persistence will ultimately be a tribute to those consumers who have endorsed the philosophy to ensure that it becomes a permanent part of good practice.

References

Ackerson, B. J., & Harrison, W. D. (2000). Practitioners' perceptions of empowerment. *Families in Society, 81*(3), 238–244.

Across Boundaries. (2012). www.acrossboundaries.ca/index.html

Adams, R. (1996). *Social work and empowerment.* London: Macmillan.

Advancing Futures for Adults with Autism (AFAA). (2011). www.afaa-us.org

Akshoomoff, N. (2006). Autism spectrum disorders: Introduction. *Child Neuropsychology, 12,* 245–246.

Altman, S., Haeri, S., & Cohen, L. J. (2006). Predictors of relapse in bipolar disorder: A review. *Journal of Psychiatric Practice, 12*(5), 269–282.

American Psychiatric Association (APA). (2000). *Diagnostic and statistical manual of mental disorders* (4th ed., text revision). Washington, DC: American Psychiatric Association Press.

American Religious Identification Survey. (2009). *American Religious Identification Survey (ARIS 2008): Summary report March 2009.* http://www.scribd.com/doc/17136871/American-Religious-Identification-Survey-ARIS-2008-Summary-Report

Amering, M., & Schmolke, M. (2009). *Recovery in mental health: Reshaping scientific and clinical responsibilities.* Hoboken, NJ: Wiley Blackwell.

Anderson, R., Caputi, P., & Oades, L. (2006). Stages of recovery instrument: Development of a measure of recovery from serious mental illness. *Australian and New Zealand Journal of Psychiatry, 40,* 972–980.

Anthony, W. A. (1993). Recovery from mental illness: The guiding vision of the mental health service system in the 1990s. *Psychosocial Rehabilitation Journal, 16*(4), 11–23.

Arieti, S. (1974). *Interpretation of schizophrenia* (2nd ed.). New York: Basic Books.

Barnes, C., & Mitchell, P. (2005). Considerations in the management of bipolar disorder in women. *Australian and New Zealand Journal of Psychiatry, 39*(8), 662–673.

Barnett, J. E., Jeffrety, E., & Johnson, W. B. (2011). Integrating spirituality and religion into psychotherapy: Persistent dilemmas, ethical issues, and a proposed decision-making process. *Ethics & Behavior, 21*(2), 147–164.

Barnhill, G. (2007). Outcomes in adults with Asperger syndrome. *Focus on Autism and Other Developmental Disabilities, 22*(2), 116–126.

Barrett, B., Young, M. S., Teague, G. B., Winarski, J. T., Moore, K. A., & Ochshorn, E. (2010). Recovery orientation of treatment, consumer empowerment, and satisfaction with services: A mediatorial model. *Psychiatric Rehabilitation Journal, 34*(2), 153–156.

Basco, M. R., & Rush, A. J. (2005). *Cognitive-behavioral therapy for bipolar disorder* (2nd ed.). New York: Guilford Press.

Beasley, J. B., & Hurley, A. D. (2007). Public systems supports for people with intellectual disability and mental health needs in the United States. *Mental Health Aspects of Developmental Disabilities, 10*(3), 118–120.

Beck, A., Rush, A., Shaw, B., & Emery, G. (1979). *Cognitive therapy of depression.* New York: Guilford Press.

Beecher, B. (2009). The medical model, mental health practitioners, and individuals with schizophrenia and their families. *Journal of Social Work Practice, 23*(1), 9–20.

Benjet, C., Thompson, R. J., & Gotib, I. H. (2010). 5-HTTLPR moderates the effect of relational peer victimization on depressive symptoms in adolescent girls. *Journal of Child Psychology and Psychiatry, 51*(2), 173–179.

Bentley, K., & Walsh, J. (2006). *The social worker and psychotropic medication* (3rd ed.). Pacific Grove, CA: Brooks/Cole.

Berg, I., & Dolan, Y. (2001). *Tales of solutions: A collection of hope inspiring stories.* New York: W. W. Norton.

Berk, M., Conus, P., Lucas, N., Hallam, K., Malhi, G. S., Dodd, S., . . . McGorry, P. (2007). Setting the stage: From prodrome to treatment resistance in bipolar disorder. *Bipolar Disorders, 9,* 671–678.

Bertolino, B., & O'Hanlon, B. (2002). *Collaborative, competency-based counseling and therapy.* Boston: Allyn & Bacon.

Beutler, L. E., & Baker, M. (1998). The movement toward empirical validation: At what level should we analyze, and who are the consumers? In K. S. Dobson & K. D. Craig (Eds.), *Empirically supported therapies: Best practice in professional psychology* (pp. 43–65). Thousand Oaks, CA: Sage.

Billstedt, E., Gillberg, C., & Gillberg, C. (2005). Autism after adolescence: Population-based 13- to 22-year follow-up study of 120 individuals with autism diagnosed in childhood. *Journal of Autism and Developmental Disorders, 35*(3), 351–360.

Birmaher, B., Axelson, D., Strober, M., Gill, M. K., Valeri, S., Chiapetta, L., . . . Keller, M. (2006). Clinical course of children and adolescents with bipolar spectrum disorders. *Archives of General Psychiatry, 63*(2), 175–183.

Boehm, A., & Staples, L. H. (2002). The functions of the social worker in empowering: The voices of consumers and professionals. *Social Work, 47*(4), 449–460.

Boisen, A. (1936). *The exploration of the inner world.* Philadelphia: University of Pennsylvania Press.

Boog, B., Coenen, H., & Keune, L. (Eds.). (2001). *Action research: Empowerment and reflection.* Oisterwijk, Netherlands: Dutch University Press.

Borras, L., Mohr, S., Gillierson, C., Branndt, P., Rieben, I., Leclerc, C., & Huguelet, P. (2010). Religion and spirituality: How clinicians in Quebec and Geneva cope with the issue when faced with patients suffering from chronic psychosis. *Community Mental Health Journal, 46*(1), 77–86.

Brody, E. M., & Farber, B. A. (1996). The effects of therapist experience and consumer diagnosis on countertransference. *Psychotherapy, 33*(3), 372–380.

Bruhn, J. G., Levine, H. G., & Levine, P. L. (1993). *Managing boundaries in the helping professions.* Springfield, IL: Charles C Thomas.

Brun, C., & Rapp, C. (2001). Strengths-based case management: Individuals' perspectives on strengths and the case manager relationship. *Social Work, 46*(3), 278–288.

Cadenhead, K. S., & Braff, D. L. (2000). Information processing and attention in schizophrenia: Clinical and functional correlates and treatment of cognitive impairment. In T. Sharma & P. Harvey (Eds.), *Cognition in schizophrenia: Impairments, importance, and treatment strategies* (pp. 92–106). New York: Oxford University Press.

Calabrese, J. D., & Corrigan, P. W. (2005). Beyond dementia praecox: Findings from long-term follow-up studies of schizophrenia. In R. Ralph & P. W. Corrigan (Eds.), *Recovery in mental illness: Broadening our understanding of wellness* (pp. 63–84). Washington, DC: American Psychological Association.

Campbell, R. J. (2004). *Campbell's psychiatric dictionary* (8th ed.). New York: Oxford University Press.

Cardno, A., & Murray, R. M. (2003). The "classic" genetic epidemiology of schizophrenia. In R. M. Murray & P. B. Jones (Eds.), *The epidemiology of schizophrenia* (pp. 195–219). New York: Cambridge University Press.

Carpenter, L. L., Gawuga, C. E., Tyrka, A. R., Lee, J. K., Anderson, G. M., & Price, L. H. (2010). Association between plasma IL-6 response to acute stress and early-life adversity in healthy adults. *Neuropsychopharmacology, 35,* 2617–2623.

Carroll, M. A. (1994). Empowerment theory: Philosophical and practical difficulties. *Canadian Psychology, 35*(4), 376–381.

Caspi, A., Sudgen, K., Moffit, T. E., Taylor, A., Craig, I. W., Harrington, H., . . . Poulton, R. (2003). Influence of life stress on depression: Moderation by a polymorphism in the 5-TT gene. *Science*, July 18, 386(4).

Cederlund, M., Hagberg, B., Billstedt, E., Gillberg, I. C., & Gillberg, C. (2008). Asperger syndrome and autism: A comparative longitudinal follow-up study more than 5 years after original diagnosis. *Journal of Autism and Developmental Disorders*, 38(1), 72–85.

Centers for Disease Control and Prevention (CDC). (2012). *New data on autism spectrum disorders.* www.cdc.gov/Features/CountingAutism/

Chambless, D. L. (1998). Empirically validated treatments. In G. P. Koocher, J. C. Norcross, & S. S. Hill (Eds.), *Psychologists' desk reference* (pp. 209–219). New York: Oxford University Press.

Chue, P. (2006). The relationship between patient satisfaction and treatment outcomes in schizophrenia. *Journal of Psychopharmacology*, 38(19).

Clark, C. L. (2000). *Social work ethics: Politics, principles, and practice.* Houndmills, Basingstoke, Hampshire, UK: MacMillan Press.

Clarke, I. (Ed.). (2000). *Psychosis and spirituality: Exploring the new frontier.* London: Whurr.

Clarke, S. P., Crowe, T. P., Oades, L. G., & Deane, F. P. (2009). Do goal-setting interventions improve the quality of goals in mental health services? *Psychiatric Rehabilitation Journal*, 32(4), 292–299.

Cohen, D. (2002). Research on the drug treatment of schizophrenia: A critical reappraisal and implications for social work education. *Journal of Social Work Education*, 38(2), 217–239.

Conklin, H. M., & Iacono, W. G. (2003). At issue: Assessment of schizophrenia: Getting closer to the cause. *Schizophrenia Bulletin*, 29(3), 409–412.

Cook, J. A., Copeland, M. E., Corey, L., Buffington, E., Jonikas, J. A., Curtis, L. C., . . . Nichols, W. H. (2010). Developing the evidence base for peer-led services: Changes among participants following Wellness Recovery Action Planning (WRAP) education in two statewide initiatives. *Psychiatric Rehabilitation Journal*, 34(2), 113–120.

Cooper, J. O., Heron, T. E., & Heward, W. L. (2007). *Applied behavior analysis* (2nd ed.). Upper Saddle River, NJ: Pearson.

Copeland, M. E. (2008). *The WRAP story: First person accounts of personal and system recovery and transformation.* West Dummerton, VT: Peach Press.

Corrigan, P. W., Salzer, M., Ralph, R. O., Sangster, Y., & Keck, L. (2004). Examining the factor structure of the recovery assessment scale. *Schizophrenia Bulletin*, 30(4), 1035–1041.

Cox, M. (1997). The great feast of languages: Passwords to the psychotic's inner world. In C. Mace & F. Margison (Eds.), *Psychotherapy of psychosis* (pp. 31–48). London: Gaskell.

Cuijpers P., van Straten, A., Andersson, G., & van Oppen, P. (2008). Psychotherapy for depression in adults: A meta-analysis of comparative outcome studies. *Journal of Consulting and Clinical Psychology*, 76(6), 909–922.

Curtis, L. C., & Hodge, M. (1994). Old standards, new dilemmas: Ethics and boundaries in community support services. In *Introduction to psychiatric rehabilitation* (pp. 340–354). Columbia, MD: International Association of Psychosocial Rehabilitation Services.

Dail, H. (2010). *Recovery and consumer mental health movement.* Unpublished manuscript, School of Social Work, Virginia Commonwealth University, Richmond, VA.

Dallin, B. (1986). Art break: A 2-day expressive art therapy program using art and psychodrama to further the termination process. *The Arts in Psychotherapy*, 13, 137–142.

Davidson, L. (2003). *Living outside mental illness: Qualitative studies of recovery in schizophrenia.* New York: New York University Press.

Davidson, L., Borg, M., Marin, I., Topor, A., Mezzina, R., & Sells, D. (2005). Process of recovery in serious mental illness: Finding from a multinational study. *American Journal of Psychiatric Rehabilitation*, 8, 177–201.

Davidson, L., Flanagan, E., Roe, D., & Styron, T. (2006). Leading a horse to water: An action perspective on mental health policy. *Journal of Clinical Psychology*, 62(9), 1141–1155.

Davidson, L., Harding, C., & Spaniol, L. (Eds.). (2006). *Recovery from severe mental illness: Research evidence and implications for practice.* Boston: Center for Psychiatric Rehabilitation.

Davidson, L., O'Connell, M. J., Tondora, J., Lawless, M., & Evans, A. C. (2005). Recovery in serious mental illness: A new wine or just a new bottle? *Professional Psychology: Research and Practice, 36*(5), 480–487.

Davidson, L., O'Connell, M., Tondora, J., Styron, T., & Kangas, K. (2006). The top ten concerns about recovery encountered in mental health system transformation. *Psychiatric Services 57*(5), 640–645.

de Bruin, E. I., Ferdinand, R. F., Meester, S., de Nijs, P. F. A., & Verheij, F. (2007). *Journal of Autism and Developmental Disorders, 37,* 877–886.

Deegan, P. (1996). Recovery as a journey of the heart. *Psychiatric Rehabilitation Journal, 19*(3), 91–97.

Deegan, P. E., & Drake, R. E. (2006). Shared decision making and medication management in the recovery process. *Psychiatric Services, 57*(11), 1636–1639.

Dein, S. (2007). Seraphs and snakes: Spirituality, agency, and psychopathology. *Primary Care & Community Psychiatry, 12*(3–4), 117–121.

DeJong, P., & Berg, I. K. (2008). *Interviewing for solutions* (3rd ed.). Pacific Grove, CA: Brooks/ Cole.

Dekovic, M. (1999). Parent-adolescent conflict: Possible determinants and consequences. *International Journal of Behavioral Development, 23*(4), 977–1000.

des Portes, V., Hagerman, R. J., & Hendren, R. L. (2003). Pharmacotherapy. In S. Ozonoff, S. J. Rogers, & R. L. Hendren (Eds.), *Autism spectrum disorders: A research review for practitioners* (pp. 161–186). Washington, DC: American Psychiatric Association.

Detera-Wadleigh, S. D., & McMahon, F. J. (2006). G72/G30 in schizophrenia and bipolar disorder: Review and meta-analysis. *Biological Psychiatry, 60*(2), 106–114.

Dilks, S., Tasker, F., & Wren, B. (2008). Building bridges to observational perspectives: A grounded theory of therapy processes in psychosis. *Psychology and Psychotherapy: Theory, Research and Practice, 81,* 209–229.

Dolgoff, R., Loewenberg, F. M., & Harrington, D. (2009). *Ethical decisions for social work practice* (8th ed). Itasca, IL: F. E. Peacock.

Doreen, C. (1998). Knowing patients: How much and how well? In P. Griffiths & J. Ord (Eds.), *Face to face with distress: The professional use of self in psychosocial care* (pp. 135–146). Oxford, UK: Butterworth-Heinemann.

Dorfman, R. A. (1996). *Clinical social work: Definition, practice, and vision.* New York: Brunner/ Mazell.

Ehrenreich, J. (1985). *The altruistic imagination: A history of social work and social policy in the United States.* Ithaca, NY: Cornell University Press.

Essock, S. M., Mueser, K. T., Drake, R. E., Covell, N. H., McHugo, G. J., Frisman, L. K., . . . Swain, K. (2006). Comparison of ACT and standard case management for delivering integrated treatment of co-occurring disorders. *Psychiatric Services, 57*(2), 185–196.

Everett, J. E., Homstead, K., & Drisko, J. (2007). Frontline worker perceptions of the empowerment process in community-based agencies. *Social Work, 52*(2), 161–170.

Fallot, R. D. (1998). Assessment of spirituality and implications for service delivery. In R. D. Fallot (Ed.), *Spirituality and religion in recovery from mental illness* (Vol. 1, pp. 13–23). San Francisco: Jossey-Bass.

Fallot, R. D. (2001). Spirituality and religion in psychiatric rehabilitation and recovery from mental illness. *International Review of Psychiatry, 13,* 110–116.

Fallot, R. D., & Newburn, J. (2000). *A spiritual and trauma recovery group for women with co-occurring disorders.* Washington, DC: Community Connections.

Faravelli, C., Rosi, S., & Scarpato, M. A. (2006). Threshold and subthreshold bipolar disorders in the Sesto Fiorentino Study. *Journal of Affective Disorders, 94*(1–3), 111–119.

Farber, N. J., Novack, D. H., & O'Brient, M. K. (1997). Love, boundaries, and the patient-physician relationship. *Archives of Internal Medicine, 157*(20), 2291–2295.

Fava, G. A., Ruini, C., & Rafanelli, C. (2005). Sequential treatment of mood and anxiety disorders. *Journal of Clinical Psychiatry, 66*(11), 1392–1400.

Fergusson, D. M., Boden, J. M., & Horwood, L. J. (2008). Exposure to childhood sexual and physical abuse and adjustment in adulthood. *Child Abuse & Neglect, 32*(6), 607–619.

Findling, R. L. (2009). Treatment of childhood-onset bipolar disorder. In C. A. Zarate & H. K. Manji (Eds.), *Bipolar depression: Molecular neurobiology, clinical diagnosis and pharmacotherapy* (pp. 241–252). Cambridge, MA: Birkhäuser.

Flanders, S. C., Engelhart, L., Pandina, G. J., & McCracken, J. T. (2007). Direct health care costs for children with pervasive developmental disorders: 1996–2002. *Administration and Policy in Mental Health and Mental Health Services Research, 34*(3), 213–220.

Floersch, J. (2003). The subjective experience of youth psychotropic treatment. *Social Work in Mental Health, 1*(4), 51–69.

Fong, R., & Furuto, S. (Eds.). (2001). *Culturally competent practice: Skills, interventions, and evaluations*. Boston: Allyn & Bacon.

Frank, E. (2007). Interpersonal and social rhythm therapy: A means of improving depression and preventing relapse in bipolar disorder. *Journal of Clinical Psychology: In Session, 63*(5), 463–473.

Frank, J. D., & Frank, J. B. (1993). *Persuasion and healing: A comparative study of psychotherapy*. Baltimore: Johns Hopkins.

Frankl, V. E. (1988). *The will to meaning: Foundations and applications of logotherapy*. New York: Meridian.

Frankl, V. E. (2000). *Recollections*. New York: Persens Publishing.

Fraser, M. W. (2004). Intervention research in social work: Recent advances and continuing challenges. *Research on Social Work Practice, 14*(3), 210–222.

Frese, F. J., & Davis, W. W. (1997). The consumer-survivor movement, recovery, and consumer professionals. *Professional Psychology: Research and Practice, 28*(3), 243–245.

Fukui, S., Starnino, V. R., Susana, M., Davidson, L. J., Cook, K., Rapp, C. A., & Gowdy, E. A. (2011). Effect of Wellness Recovery Action Plan (WRAP) participation on psychiatric symptoms, sense of hope, and recovery. *Psychiatric Rehabilitation Journal, 34*(3), 214–222.

Furman, R. (2009). Ethical considerations of evidence-based practice. *Social Work, 54*(1), 82–84.

Gabbard, G. O. (1995). Countertransference: The emerging common ground. *International Journal of Psychoanalysis, 76*, 475–485.

Gabbard, G. O., & Lester, E. P. (1995). *Boundaries and boundary violations in psychoanalysis*. New York: Basic Books.

Gadow, K., DeVincent, C., & Schneider, J. (2008). Predictors of psychiatric symptoms in children with an autism spectrum disorder. *Journal of Autism and Developmental Disorders, 38*(9), 1710–1720.

Geller, B., Tillman, R., Bolhofner, K., & Zimerman, B. (2008). Child bipolar I disorder: Prospective continuity with adult bipolar I disorder; characteristics of second and third episodes; predictors of 8-year outcome. *Archives of General Psychiatry, 65*(10), 1125–1133.

Goldstein, E. G. (1995). *Ego psychology and social work practice* (2nd ed.). New York: Free Press.

Goldstein, E. G., Miehls, D., & Ringel, S. (2009). *Advanced clinical social work: Relational principles and techniques*. New York: Columbia University Press.

Goodman, S. H. (2007). Depression in mothers. *Annual Review of Clinical Psychology, 3*, 107–135.

Goss, J. (2006). The poetics of bipolar disorder. *Pragmatics & Cognition, 14*(1), 83–110.

Grant, B. F., Stinson, F. S., Hasin, D. S., Dawson, D. A., Chou, S. P., Ruan, W. J., & Huang, B. (2005). Prevalence, correlates, and comorbidity of bipolar I disorder and axis I and II disorder: Results from the national epidemiological survey on alcohol and related conditions. *Journal of Clinical Psychiatry, 66*, 1205–1215.

Gutheil, I. A. (1993). Rituals and termination procedures. *Smith College Studies in Social Work, 63*(2), 163–176.

Gutheil, T. G., & Gabbard, G. O. (1998). Misuses and misunderstandings of boundary theory in clinical and regulatory settings. *American Journal of Psychiatry, 155*(3), 409–414.

Gutman, L. M., & Sameroff, A. J. (2004). Continuities in depression from adolescence to young adulthood: Contrasting ecological influences. *Development and Psychopathology, 16*, 967–984.

Hamrin, V., & Pachler, M. (2007). Pediatric bipolar disorder: Evidence-based psychopharmacological treatments. *Journal of Child and Adolescent Psychiatric Nursing, 20*(1), 40–58.

Hanson, E., Kalish, L. A., Bunce, E., Curtis, C., McDaniel, S., Ware, J., & Petry, J. (2007). Use of complementary and alternative medicine among children diagnosed with autism spectrum disorder. *Journal of Autism and Developmental Disorders, 37*(4), 628–636.

Harper, K., & Lantz, J. (2007). *Cross-cultural practice: Social work with diverse populations* (2nd ed.). Chicago: Lyceum Books.

Harrigan, M. P., Fauri, D. P., & Netting, F. E. (1998). Termination: Expanding the concept for macro social work practice. *Journal of Sociology and Social Welfare, 25*(4), 61–80.

Harrington, J., Rosen, L., Garnecho, A., & Patrick, P. (2006). Parental perceptions and use of complementary and alternative medicine practices for children with autistic spectrum disorders in private practice. *Journal of Developmental and Behavioral Pediatrics, 27*(Suppl. 2), S156–161.

Harris, M., & Bergman, H. C. (1988). Clinical case management for the chronically mentally ill: A conceptual analysis. In M. Harris, & L. Bachrach (Eds.), *Clinical case management* (pp. 5–13). New Directions for Mental Health Services, 40. San Francisco: Jossey-Bass.

Harvey, P. D. (2000). Formal thought disorder in schizophrenia: Characteristics and cognitive underpinnings. In T. Sharma & P. Harvey (Eds.), *Cognition in schizophrenia: Impairments, importance, and treatment strategies* (pp. 107–125). New York: Oxford University Press.

Hassan, S., Cinq-Mars, C., & Sigman, M. (2000). Conflict in group therapy of chronic schizophrenics: Coping with aggression. *American Journal of Psychotherapy, 54*(2), 243–255.

Havens, L. L. (1996). *A safe place: Laying the groundwork of psychotherapy.* Cambridge, MA: Harvard University Press, 1989.

Hayes, J. A., Gelso, C. J., & Hummel, A. M. (2011). Managing countertransference. *Psychotherapy, 48*(1), 88–97.

Helgeson, V., Reynolds, K., & Tomich, P. (2006). A meta-analytic review of benefit finding and growth. *Journal of Consulting and Clinical Psychology, 74*, 797–816.

Herlihy, B., & Corey, G. (1997). *Boundary issues in counseling: Multiple roles and responsibilities.* Alexandria, VA: American Counseling Association.

Hermansson, G. (1997). Boundaries and boundary management in counseling: The never-ending story. *British Journal of Guidance and Counseling, 25*(2), 133–146.

Hewitt, J., & Coffey, M. (2005). Therapeutic working relationships with people with schizophrenia: Literature review. *Journal of Advanced Nursing, 52*(5), 561–570.

Hirschfeld, R. M. A., Lewis, L., & Vornik, L. A. (2003). Perceptions and impact of bipolar disorder: How far have we come? Results of the National Depressive and Manic Depressive Association's 2000 survey of individuals with bipolar disorder. *Journal of Clinical Psychiatry, 64*(2), 161–174.

Holford, N. L. (1982). Religious ideation in schizophrenia. *Dissertation Abstracts International, 43*(6-B), 1983-B.

Holmes, J. (1997). "Too early, too late": Endings in psychotherapy—An attachment perspective. *British Journal of Psychotherapy, 14*(2), 159–171.

Holter, M. (2004). Autistic spectrum disorders: Assessment and intervention. In P. Allen-Meares & M. Fraser (Eds.), *Intervention with children and adolescents: An interdisciplinary perspective* (pp. 205–228). Washington, DC: National Association of Social Workers Press.

Howlin, P. (2005). Outcomes in autism spectrum disorders. In F. R. Volkmar, R. Paul, A. Klin, & D. Cohen (Eds.), *Handbook of autism and pervasive developmental disorders: Vol. 1. Diagnosis, development, neurobiology, and behavior* (3rd ed.) (pp. 201–220). Hoboken, NJ: John Wiley.

Huang, X., Lei, Z., & El-Mallach, R. S. (2007). Lithium normalizes elevated intracellular sodium. *Bipolar Disorder, 9*(3), 298–300.

Huguelet, P., Mohr, S., Borras, L., Gillierson, C., & Brandt (2006). Spirituality and religious practices among outpatients with schizophrenia and their clinicians. *Psychiatric Services, 57*(3), 366–372.

Imbrie, G. S. (1985). Untwisting the illusion. *Journal of Orthomolecular Psychiatry, 14,* 143–145.

Institute of Medicine. (2004). *Immunization safety review: Vaccines and autism.* http://www .nap.edu/catalog.php?record_id=10997#description

Ivleva, E., Thaker, G., & Tamminga, C. A. (2008). Comparing genes and phenomenology in the major psychoses: Schizophrenia and bipolar I disorder. *Schizophrenia Bulletin, 34*(4), 734–742.

Jackson, R. L. (2001). *The clubhouse model: Empowering applications of theory to generalist practice.* Pacific Grove, CA: Brooks/Cole.

Jacobs, T. J. (1999). Countertransference past and present: A review of the concept. *International Journal of Psychoanalysis, 80,* 575–594.

Jacobson N., & Greenley. D. (2001). What is recovery? A conceptual model and explication. *Psychiatric Services, 52*(4), 482–485.

Jerrell, J. M., Cousins, V. C., & Roberts, K. M. (2006). Psychometrics of the Recovery Process Inventory. *Journal of Behavioral Health Services & Research, 33*(4), 464–474.

Jesner, O. S., Aref-Adib, M., & Coren, E. (2007). Risperidone for autism spectrum disorder. *Cochrane Database of Systematic Reviews, 1,* Art. No. CD005040.

Joiner, T. E., Orden, K. A., Witte, T. K., & Rudd, M. D. (2009). Diagnoses associated with suicide. In T. E. Joiner, V. Orden, K. A. Witte, T. K. Rudd, & M. David (Eds.), *The interpersonal theory of suicide: Guidance for working with suicidal clients* (pp. 21–51). Washington, DC: American Psychological Association.

Kanas, N. (2005). Evidential support for the value of integrative group therapy for patients with schizophrenia. *Directions in Psychiatry, 25*(3), 231–239.

Kanter, J. (Ed.). (1995). *Clinical issues in case management.* San Francisco: Jossey-Bass.

Kanter, J. (1996). Case management with longterm patients. In S. M. Soreff (Ed.), *Handbook for the treatment of the seriously mentally ill* (pp. 259–275). Seattle: Hogrefe & Huber.

Kanter, J. (2006). Clinical case management, case management, and ACT. *Psychiatric Services, 57*(4), 578–579.

Karasu, T. B., Gelenberg, A., Merriam, A., & Wang, P. (2002). Practice guidelines for the treatment of patients with major depressive disorder. In *American Psychiatric Association practice guidelines for the treatment of psychiatric disorder: Compendium 2002* (2nd ed.) (pp. 463–545). Washington, DC: American Psychiatric Publishing.

Karls, J. M., & Wandrei, K. E. (Eds.). (1994). *Person-in-environment system: The PIE classification system for social functioning problems.* Washington, DC: National Association of Social Workers Press.

Karp, D. A. (1995). *Speaking of sadness.* New York: Oxford.

Keefe, R. S. E. (2000). Working memory dysfunction and its relevance to schizophrenia. In T. Sharma & P. Harvey (Eds.), *Cognition in schizophrenia: Impairments, importance, and treatment strategies* (pp. 16–50). New York: Oxford University Press.

Kehoe, N. C. (1998). Religious-issues group therapy. In R. D. Fallot (Ed.), *Spirituality and religion in recovery from mental illness* (Vol. 80, pp. 45–55). San Francisco: Jossey-Bass.

Kessler, R. C., Berglund, P., Demler, O., Jin, R., Merikangas, K. R., & Walters, E. E. (2005). Lifetime prevalence and age-of-onset distributions of DSM-IV disorders on the National Comorbidity Survey Replication. *Archives of General Psychiatry, 62*(6), 593–602.

Kessler, R. C., Chiu, W. T., Demler, O., & Walters, E. E. (2005). Prevalence, severity, and comorbidity of 12-month *DSM-IV* disorders in the National Comorbidity Survey Replication. *Archives of General Psychiatry, 62*(6), 617–627.

Ketter, T. A., & Wang, P. O. (2010). Overview of pharmacotherapy for bipolar disorders. In T. A. Ketter (Ed.), *Handbook of diagnosis and treatment of bipolar disorders* (pp. 83–106). Arlington, VA: American Psychiatric Publishing.

Kidd, S. A., George, L., O'Connell, M., Sylvestre, J., Kirkpatrick, H., Browne, G., . . . Davidson, L. (2011). Recovery-oriented service provision and clinical outcomes in assertive community treatment. *Psychiatric Rehabilitation Journal, 34*(3), 194–201.

Kirsch, B., & Cockburn, L. (2009). The Canadian occupational performance measure: A tool for recovery-based practice. *Psychiatric Rehabilitation Journal, 32*(3), 171–176.

Knapp, H. (2003). Countertransference issues in concurrent therapy with a schizophrenic individual. *Psychoanalysis & Psychotherapy, 20*(1), 45–66.

Kocan, M. (1988). *Transference and countertransference in clinical work.* Dayton, MD: American Healthcare Institute.

Koenig, H. G., & Pritchett, J. (1998). Religion and psychotherapy. In H. G. Koenig (Ed.), *Handbook of religion and mental health* (pp. 323–336). San Diego, CA: Academic Press.

Koyama, T., Tachimor, H., & Osada, H. (2006). Cognitive and symptom profiles in high-functioning pervasive developmental disorder not otherwise specified and attention-deficit/hyperactivity disorder. *Journal of Autism and Developmental Disorders, 36*(3), 373–380.

Kraaij, V., Arensman, E., & Spinhoven, P. (2002). Negative life events and depression in elderly persons: A meta-analysis. *Journals of Gerontology Series B-Psychological Sciences & Social Sciences, 57B*(1), 87–94.

Krill, D. F. (1996). Existential social work. In F. J. Turner (Ed.), *Social work treatment* (4th ed.) (pp. 250–281). New York: Free Press.

Kuipers, E., Garety, P., Fowler, D., . . . Bebbington, P. (2006). Cognitive, emotional, and social processes in psychosis: Refining cognitive behavioral therapy for persistent positive symptoms. *Schizophrenia Bullentin, 32*(Suppl. 1), S24–S31.

Kumsta, R., Stevens, S., Brookes, K., Schlotz, W., Castle, J., Beckett, C., . . . Sonuga-Barke, E. (2010). 5HTT genotype moderates the influence of early institutional deprivation on emotional problems in adolescence: Evidence from the English and Romanian Adoptee (ERA) Study. *Journal of Child Psychology and Psychiatry, 51*(7), 755–762.

Lantz, J. (1978). *Family and marital therapy.* New York: Appleton-Century-Crofts.

Lantz, J. (2002). Existential psychotherapy: What endures? *Voices, 38*, 28–33.

Lantz, J., & Gregoire, T. (2000). Existential psychotherapy with Vietnam veteran couples: A twenty-five year report. *Contemporary Family Therapy, 22*, 19–37.

Larson, G. (2008). Anti-oppressive practice in mental health. *Journal of Progressive Social Services, 19*(1), 39–53.

Latimer, E. A., Bond, G. R., & Drake, R. E. (2011). Economic approaches to improving access to evidence-based and recovery-oriented services for people with severe mental illness. *The Canadian Journal of Psychiatry, 56*(9), 523–528.

Lawrence, R., Bradshaw, T., & Mairs, H. (2006). Group cognitive behavioral therapy for schizophrenia: A systematic review of the literature. *Journal of Psychiatric and Mental Health Nursing, 13*(6), 673–681.

Lazarus, R. S., & Lazarus, B. N. (1994). *Passion and reason: Making sense of our emotions.* New York: Oxford.

Leahy, R. L. (2007). Bipolar disorder: Causes, contexts, and treatments. *Journal of Clinical Psychology, 63*(5), 417–424.

Lee, J. A. B. (2001). *The empowerment approach to social work practice: Building the beloved community* (2nd ed.). New York: Columbia University Press.

Lee, M. Y., & Greene, G. J. (2003). A teaching framework for transformative multicultural social work education. *Journal of Ethnic & Cultural Diversity in Social Work: Innovation in Theory, Research & Practice, 12*(3), 1–28.

Lemstra, M., Neudorf, C., D'Arcy, C., Kunst, A., Warren, L. M., & Bennett, N. R. (2008). A systematic review of depressed mood and anxiety by SES in youth aged 10–15 years. *Canadian Journal of Public Health, 99*(2), 125–129.

Leonardson, D. (2007). Empowerment in social work: An individual versus a relational perspective. *International Journal of Social Welfare, 16*(1), 3–11.

Leskovec, T. J., Rowles, B. M., & Findlay, R. L. (2008). Pharmacological treatment options for autism spectrum disorders in children and adolescents. *Harvard Review of Psychiatry, 16*(2), 97–112.

Liberman, R. P. (2008). *Recovery from disability: Manual of psychiatric rehabilitation.* Arlington, VA: American Psychiatric Publishing.

Lieberman, J., Stroup, S., McEvoy, J., Swartz, M., Rosenheck, R., Perkins, D., . . . Hsiao, J. (2005). Effectiveness of antipsychotic drugs in patients with chronic schizophrenia. *New England Journal of Medicine, 353,* 1209–1223.

Lindgren, K. N., & Coursey, R. D. (1995). Spirituality and serious mental illness: A two-part study. *Psychosocial Rehabilitation Journal, 18*(3), 93–111.

Liptak, G. S., Stuart, T., & Auinger, P. (2006). Health care utilization and expenditures for children with autism: Data from U.S. national samples. *Journal of Autism and Developmental Disabilities, 36*(3), 871–879.

Longhofer, J., Kubek, P. M., & Floersch, J. (2010). *On being and having a case manager: A relational approach to recovery in mental health.* New York: Columbia University Press.

Loveland, D., Randall, K. W., & Corrigan, P. W. (2005). Research methods for exploring and assessing recovery. In R. O. Ralph & P. W. Corrigan (Eds.), *Recovery in mental illness: Broadening our understanding of wellness* (pp. 19–59). Washington, DC: American Psychological Association.

Lukoff, D. (2005). Spiritual and transpersonal approaches to psychotic disorders. In S. G. Mijares & G. S. Khalsa (Eds.), *The psychospiritual clinician's handbook: Alternative methods for understanding and treating mental disorders* (pp. 233–257). New York: Haworth Press.

Lysaker, P. H., Buck, K. D., & Lintner, J. I. (2009). Addressing recovery from severe mental illness in clinical supervision of advanced students. *Journal of Psychosocial Nursing, 47*(4), 36–42.

Maimberg, R. D., & Vaeth, M. (2006). Perinatal risk factors and infantile autism. *Acta Psychiatrica Scandinavica, 114,* 257–264.

Malmberg, L., & Fenton, M. (2005). Individual psychodynamic psychotherapy and psychoanalysis for schizophrenia and severe mental illness. *The Cochrane Database of Systematic Reviews, 4,* Art. No. CD001360.

Mandell, D. (2008). Power, care, and vulnerability: Considering use of self in child welfare work. *Journal of Social Work Practice, 22*(2), 235–248.

Mandell, D. S., Novak, M., & Zubritsky, L. (2005). The role of culture in families' treatment decisions for children with autism spectrum disorders. *Mental Retardation and Developmental Disabilities Research Reviews, 11*(2), 110–115.

Marangell, L. B., Kupfer, D. J., Sachs, G. S., & Swann, A. C. (2006). Emerging therapies for bipolar depression. *Journal of Clinical Psychiatry, 67*(7), 1140–1151.

Marecek, J. (2006). Social suffering, gender, and women's depression. In C. L. M. Keyes & S. H. Goodman (Eds.), *Women and depression: Handbook for the social, behavioral, and biomedical sciences* (pp. 283–308). New York: Cambridge University Press.

Marshall, S. L., Oades, L. G., & Crowe, T. P. (2009). Mental health consumers' perceptions of receiving recovery-focused services. *Journal of Evaluation in Clinical Practice, 15*(4), 654–659.

Masterson, S., & Owen, S. (2006). Mental health service user's social and individual empowerment: Using theories of power to elucidate far-reaching strategies. *Journal of Mental Health, 15*(1), 19–34.

Matza, L. S., Rajagopalan, K. S., Thompson, C. L., & Lissovoy, G. (2005). Misdiagnosed patients with bipolar disorder: Comorbidities, treatment patterns, and direct treatment costs. *Journal of Clinical Psychiatry, 66*(11), 1432–1440.

May, R., & Yalom, I. (2000). Existential psychotherapy. In R. J. Corsini & D. Wedding (Eds.), *Current psychotherapies* (5th ed.), (pp. 262–292). Itasca, IL: F. E. Peacock.

McGovern, C. W., & Sigman, M. (2005). Continuity and change from early childhood to adolescence in autism. *Journal of Child Psychology and Psychiatry, 46*(4), 401–408.

McGuffin, P., Rijsdijk, F., Andrew, M., Sham, P., Katz, R., & Cardino, A. (2003). The heritability of bipolar affective disorder and the genetic relationship to unipolar depression. *Archives of General Psychiatry, 60*, 497–502.

McLeod, B. D., Weisz, J. R., & Wood, J. J. (2007). Examining the association between parenting and childhood depression: A meta-analysis. *Clinical Psychology Review, 27*(8), 986–1003.

Mechanic, D. (2008). *Mental health and social policy: Beyond managed care* (5th ed.). Boston: Pearson.

Melvin, C. L., Carey, T. S., Goodman, F., Oldham, J. M., Williams, J. W., & Ranney, L. H. (2008). Effectiveness of antiepileptic drugs for the treatment of bipolar disorder: Findings from a systematic review. *Journal of Psychiatric Practice, 14*(1), 9–14.

Merriam-Webster's Online Dictionary. (2010). http://www.merriam-webster.com/dictionary/recovery

Miklowitz, D. J., & Otto, M. W. (2006). New psychosocial interventions for bipolar disorder: A review of literature and introduction of the systematic treatment enhancement program. *Journal of Cognitive Psychotherapy, 20*(2), 215–230.

Miklowitz, D. J., Otto, M. W., & Frank, E. (2007). Psychosocial treatments for bipolar depression: A 1-year randomized trial from the Systematic Treatment Enhancement Program. *Archives of General Psychiatry, 64*(4), 419–427.

Miklowitz, D. J., Wisniewski, S. M., Miyahara, S., Otto, M. W., & Sachs, G. S. (2005). Perceived criticism from family members as a predictor of the one-year course of bipolar disorder. *Psychiatry Research, 136*(2–3), 101–111.

Miller, S. D., Duncan, B. L., & Hubble, M. A. (2005). Outcome-informed clinical work. In J. C. Norcross & M. R. Goldfried (Eds.), *Handbook of psychotherapy integration* (2nd ed.) (pp. 84–102). New York: Oxford University Press.

Mohr, S., Borras, L., Rieben, I., Betrisey, C., Gilleron, C., Brandt, P., . . . Huguelet, P. (2010). Evolution of spirituality and religiousness in chronic schizophrenia or schizo-affective disorders: A 3-year follow-up study. *Social Psychiatry & Psychiatric Epidemiology, 45*(11), 1095–1103.

Moreno, C., Laje, G., Blanco, C., Jiung, H., Schmidt, A. B., & Olfson, M. (2007). National trends in the outpatient diagnosis and treatment of bipolar disorder in youth. *Archives of General Psychiatry, 64*(9), 1032–1038.

Mueser, K. T., Meyer, P. S., Penn, D. L., Clancy, R., Clancy, D. M., & Salyers, M. P. (2006). The Illness Management and Recovery Program: Rationale, development, and preliminary findings. *Schizophrenia Bulletin, 32*(1), S32-S43.

Murphy, M. A. (2000). Coping with the spiritual meaning of psychosis. *Psychiatric Rehabilitation Journal, 24*(2), 179–183.

Murray, R. M., Jones, P. B., & Susser, E. (2003).*The epidemiology of schizophrenia.* New York: Cambridge University Press.

National Association of Social Workers (NASW). (2008). *Code of Ethics of the National Association of Social Workers.* Washington, DC: National Association of Social Workers Press.

National Association of State Mental Health Program Directors (2012). *Tools in development: Measuring recovery at the individual, program, and system levels.* www.nasmhpd.org/spec_e-report_fall04measures.cfm

National Institute of Mental Health (NIMH). (2007). *Autism spectrum disorders: Pervasive developmental disorders.* Washington, DC: Author.

National Institute of Mental Health (NIMH). (2012). Statistics. http://www.nimh.nih.gov/statistics/index.shtml

Nelson, G., Ochocka, J., Janzen, R., & Trainor, J. (2006). A longitudinal study of mental health consumer/survivor initiatives, Part 1—Literature review and overview of the study. *Journal of Community Psychology, 34*(3), 247–260.

Neugeboren, B. (1996). *Environmental practice in the human services.* New York: Haworth.

Newman, C. F. (2006). Bipolar disorder. In F. Andrasik (Ed.), *Comprehensive handbook of personality and psychopathology: Vol. 2. Adult psychopathology* (pp. 244–261). Hoboken, NJ: John Wiley.

Newman, C. F., Leahy, R. L., Beck, A. T., Reilly-Harrington, N. A., & Gyulai, L. (2002). *Bipolar disorder: A cognitive therapy approach.* Washington, DC: American Psychological Association.

Nolen-Hoeksema, S. (2002). Gender differences in depression. In I. H. Gotlib & C. Hammen (Eds.), *Handbook of depression* (pp. 492–509). New York: Guilford Press.

Norcross, J. C., & Wampold, B. E. (2011). Evidence-based therapy relationships: Research conclusions and clinical practices. *Psychotherapy, 48*(1), 98–102.

Northway, R. (2005). Case management, care coordination, and managed care. In W. M. Nehring (Ed.), *Health promotion for persons with intellectual and developmental disabilities: The state of scientific evidence* (pp. 235–263). Washington, DC: American Association on Mental Retardation.

O'Neill, J. V. (2004). New diagnosis framework: NASW involved in setting codes for functioning. *NASW News, 49*(1), 9.

Oades, L., Deane, F., Crowe, T., Lambert, W. G., Kavanagh, D., & Lloyd, C. (2005). Collaborative recovery: An integrative model for working with individuals who experience chronic and recurring mental illness. *Australian Psychiatry, 13*(3), 279–284.

Ohio Department of Mental Health (ODMH). (2011). Recovery. http://www.mh.state.oh.us/what-we-believe/recovery/

Olfson, M., & Marcus, S. C. (2009). National patterns in antidepressant medication treatment. *Archives of General Psychiatry, 66*(8), 848–856.

Olfson, M., Blanco, C., Liu, L., Moreno, C., & Laje, G. (2006). National trends in the outpatient treatment of children and adolescents with antipsychotic drugs. *Archives of General Psychiatry, 63,* 679–685.

Onken, S. J., Craig, C. M., Ridgway, P., Ralph, R. O., & Cook, J. A. (2007). An analysis of the definitions and elements of recovery: A review of the literature. *Psychiatric Rehabilitation Journal, 31*(1), 9–22.

Oswald, D. P., & Sonenklar, N. A. (2007). Medication use among children with autism-spectrum disorders. *Journal of Child and Adolescent Psychopharmacology, 17*(3), 348–355.

Oxford Online Dictionary. (2012). http://www.websters-online-dictionary.com/definition/recovery

Padilla-Walker, L. M., Harper, J. M., & Jensen, A. C. (2010). Self-regulation as a mediator between sibling relationship quality and early adolescents' positive and negative outcomes. *Journal of Family Psychology, 24*(4), 419–428.

Palmer, B. W., & Heaton, R. K. (2000). Executive dysfunction in schizophrenia. In T. Sharma & P. Harvey (Eds.), *Cognition in schizophrenia: Impairments, importance, and treatment strategies* (pp. 51–72). New York: Oxford University Press.

Parsons, R. J. (1991). Empowerment: Purpose and practice principles in social work. *Social Work with Groups, 14*(2), 7–21.

Peliosa, L., & Lund, S. (2001). A selective overview of issues on classification, causation, and early intensive behavioral intervention for autism. *Behavior Modification, 25*(5), 678–697.

Penza, K., Heim, C., & Nemeroff, C. (2006). Trauma and depression. In C. L. M. Keyes & S. H. Goodman (Eds.), *Women and depression: Handbook for the social, behavioral, and biomedical sciences* (pp. 360–381). New York: Cambridge University Press.

Peters, E. (2001). Are delusions on a continuum? The case of religious and delusional beliefs. In I. Clarke (Ed.), *Psychosis and spirituality: Exploring the new frontier* (pp. 191–207). Philadelphia: Whurr.

Petronio, S., Ellemers, N., Giles, H., & Gallois, C. (1998). (Mis) communicating across boundaries: Interpersonal and intergroup considerations. *Communication Research, 25*(6), 571–595.

Pharoah, F. M., Rathbone, J., Mari, J. J., & Streiner, D. (2003). Family intervention for schizophrenia. *Cochrane Database of Systematic Reviews, 3*, Art. No. CD000088.

Philip, C. E. (1994). Letting go: Problems with termination when a therapist is seriously ill or dying. *Smith College Studies in Social Work, 64*(2), 169–179.

Phillips, L. J., Francey, S. M., Edwards, J., & McMurray, N. (2007). Stress and psychosis: Towards the development of new models of investigation. *Clinical Psychology Review, 27*(3), 307–317.

Piat, M., & Sabetti, J. (2009). The development of a recovery-oriented mental health system in Canada: What the experience of Commonwealth countries tells us. *Canadian Journal of Community Mental Health, 28*(2), 17–33.

Pollard, J., Hawkins, D., & Arthur, M. (1999). Risk and protection: Are both necessary to understand diverse behavioral outcomes in adolescence? *Social Work Research, 23*, 145–158.

Post, L. M. (1982). A study of the dilemmas involved in work with schizophrenic consumers. *Psychotherapy: Theory, Research, and Practice, 19*(2), 205–218.

Post, R. M., Leverich, G. B., King, Q., & Weiss, S. R. (2001). Developmental vulnerabilities to the onset and course of bipolar disorder. *Development and Psychopathology, 13*(1), 581–598.

Prochaska, J. O., & DiClemente, C. C. (1982). Transtheoretical therapy: Toward a more integrative model of change. *Psychotherapy: Theory, Research, & Practice, 19*(3), 276–288.

Ramon, S., Shera, W., Healy, B., Lachman, M., & Renouf, N. (2009). The rediscovered concept of recovery in mental illness: A multicountry comparison of policy and practice. *International Journal of Mental Health, 38*(2), 106–126.

Rapp, C. A., & Goscha, R. J. (2008). *Strengths based case management.* New York: Guilford Press.

Regehr, C., & Glancy, G. (2010). *Mental health social work practice in Canada.* Ontario, Canada: Oxford University Press.

Reindal, S. M. (2008). A social relational model of disability: A theoretical framework for special needs education? *European Journal of Special Needs Education, 23*(2), 135–146.

Rhodes, J., & Jakes, S. (2009). *Narrative CBT for psychosis.* New York: Routledge.

Roberts, A. R. (Ed.). (2009). *Social workers' desk reference* (2nd ed.). New York: Oxford University Press.

Roberts, G. A. (1997). Meaning and madness: A narrative approach to psychopathology and treatment. In C. Mace & F. Margison (Eds.), *Psychotherapy of psychosis* (pp. 255–271). London: Gaskell.

Roe, D., Hasson-Ohayon, I., Salyers, M. P., & Kravetz, S. (2009). A one-year follow-up of illness management and recovery: Participants' accounts of its impact and uniqueness. *Psychiatric Rehabilitation Journal, 32*(4), 285–291.

Rogers, S. J., & Vismara, L. A. (2008). Evidence-based comprehensive treatments for early autism. *Journal of Clinical Child and Adolescent Psychology, 37*(1), 8–38.

Rose, S. M. (1990). Advocacy/empowerment: An approach to clinical practice for social work. *Journal of Sociology and Social Welfare, 17*(2), 41–51.

Rosenthal, R. N. (2004). Overview of evidence-based practice. In A. R. Roberts & K. R. Yeager (Eds.), *Evidence-based practice manual* (pp. 20–29). New York: Oxford University Press.

Rouse, T. P. (1996). Conditions for a successful status elevation ceremony. *Deviant Behavior, 17*(1), 21–42.

Ruble, L. A., Heflinger, C. A., Renfrew, J. W., & Saunders, R. C. (2005). Access and service use by children with autism spectrum disorders in Medicaid managed care. *Journal of Autism and Developmental Disabilities, 35*(3), 3–13.

Russinova, Z., & Cash, D. (2007). Personal perspectives about the meaning of religion and spirituality among persons with serious mental illnesses. *Psychiatric Rehabilitation Journal, 30*(4), 271–284.

Russinova, Z., Prout, T. A., Wewiorski, N., Cash, D., Stepas, K. A., & Lyass, A. (2009). Use of prayer by persons with serious mental illnesses: Patterns and perceived benefits. *Counseling and Spirituality, 28*(2), 59–82.

Sackett, D. L., Richardson, W. S., Rosenberg, W., & Haynes, R. B. (1997). *Evidence-based medicine—How to practice and teach EBM.* New York: Churchill Livingstone.

Saleebey, D. (2008). The strengths perspective: Putting possibility and hope to work in our practice. In B. W. White, K. M. Sowers, & C. Dulmus (Eds.), *Comprehensive handbook of social
work and social welfare volume 1: The profession of social work* (pp. 123–142). Hoboken, NJ:
John Wiley & Sons.

Salyers, M. P., Godfrey, J. L., McGuire, A. B., Gearhart, T., Rollins, A. L., & Boyle, C. (2009).
Implementing the illness management and recovery program for consumers with severe
mental illness. *Psychiatric Services, 60*(4), 483–490.

Salyers, M. P., Hicks, L. J., & McGuire, A. B. (2009). A pilot to enhance the recovery orientation
of assertive community treatment through peer-provided illness management and
recovery. *American Journal of Psychiatric Rehabilitation, 12*(3), 191–204.

Sanville, J. (1982). Partings and impartings: Toward a nonmedical approach to interruptions
and terminations. *Clinical Social Work Journal, 10*(2), 123–131.

Savage, C. (1987). Countertransference in the therapy of schizophrenics. In E. Slakter (Ed.),
Countertransference (pp. 115–130). Northvale, NJ: Jason Aronson.

Schenkel, L. S., West, A. E., Harral, E. M., Patel, N. B., & Pavuluri, M. N. (2008). Parent-child
interactions in pediatric bipolar disorder. *Journal of Clinical Psychology, 64*(4), 422–437.

Schoenwolf, G. (1993). *Counterresistance: The therapist's interference with the therapeutic
process.* Northvale, NJ: Jason Aronson.

Schreibman, L., Stahmer, A. C., & Akshoomoff, N. (2006). Pervasive developmental disorders.
In *Clinical handbook of child behavioral assessment* (pp. 503–524). San Diego: Elsevier
Academic Press.

Schwartz, R. C., Smith, S. D., & Chopko, C. (2007). Psychotherapists' countertransference reactions toward consumers with antisocial personality disorder and schizophrenia: An
empirical test of theory. *American Journal of Psychotherapy, 61*(4), 375–393.

Seida, J. K., Ospina, M. B., Karkhaneh, M., Hartling, L., Smith, V., & Clark, B. (2009). Systematic reviews of psychosocial interventions for autism: An umbrella review. *Developmental Medicine & Child Neurology, 51*(2), 95–104.

Selten, J. P., Cantor-Craae, E., & Kahn, R. S. (2007). Migration and schizophrenia. *Current
Opinion in Psychiatry, 20*(2), 111–115.

Semrad, E. V. (1955). Psychotherapy of psychoses: An attempt at a working formulation of
some of the clinical psychopathological factors observed in schizophrenic consumers.
Journal of Clinical & Experimental Psychopathology, 16, 10–21.

Shattuck, P. T., & Grosse, S. D. (2007). Issues related to the diagnosis and treatment of autism
spectrum disorders. *Mental Retardation and Developmental Disabilities, 13*, 129–135.

Sheridan, M. J. (2008). The spiritual person. In E. D. Huchison, *Dimensions of human behavior*
(3rd ed.) (pp. 183–224). Los Angeles: Sage.

Sheridan, M. J., & Bullis, R. K. (1991). Practitioners' views of religion and spirituality: A qualitative study. *Spirituality and Social Work Journal, 2*(2), 2–10.

Sheridan, M. J., Bullis, R. K., Adcock, C. R., Berlin, S. D., & Miller, P. C. (1992). Practitioners'
personal and professional attitudes and behaviors toward religion and spirituality: Issues
for education and practice. *Journal of Social Work Education, 28*, 190–203.

Sierra, P., Livianos, L., Arques, S., Castello, J., & Rojo, L. (2007). Prodromal symptoms to relapse
in bipolar disorder. *Australian and New Zealand Journal of Psychiatry, 41*, 385–391.

Simon, R. I., & Williams, I. C. (1999). Maintaining treatment boundaries in small communities and rural areas. *Psychiatric Services, 50*(11), 1440–1446.

Skovholt, T. M. (2001). *The resilient practitioner: Burnout prevention and self-care strategies for
counselors, therapists, teachers, and health professionals.* Boston: Allyn & Bacon.

Smith, T., Magyar, C., & Arnold-Saritepe, A. (2002). *Autism spectrum disorder.* New York: John
Wiley & Sons.

Smokowski, P. R., Mann, E. A., Reynolds, A. J., & Fraser, M. (2004). Childhood risk and protective factors and late adolescent adjustment in inner city minority youth. *Children and
Youth Services Review, 26*(1), 63–91.

Spaulding, W., & Nolting, J. (2006). Psychotherapy for schizophrenia in the year 2030: Prognosis and prognostication. *Schizophrenia Bulletin, 32*(Suppl. 1), S94–S105.

Stanhope, V., Solomon, P., Finley, L., Pernell-Arnold, A., Bourjolly, J. N., & Sands, R. (2008). Evaluating the impact of cultural competency trainings from the perspective of people in recovery. *American Journal of Psychiatric Rehabilitation, 11,* 356–372.

Stone, M. H. (2006). Relationship of borderline personality disorder and bipolar disorder. *American Journal of Psychiatry, 163*(7), 1126–1128.

Stotland, N. L., Mattson, M. G., & Bergeson, S. (2008). The recovery concept: Clinician and consumer perspectives. *Journal of Psychiatric Practice, 14*(Suppl. 2), 45–54.

Strean, H. (2002). A therapist's life-threatening disease: Its impact on countertransference reactions and treatment techniques. *Psychoanalytic Inquiry, 22*(4), 559–579.

Substance Abuse and Mental Health Services Administration (SAMHSA). (2006). *SAMHSA issues consensus statement on mental health recovery.* Washington, DC. http://www.samhsa .gov/news/newsreleases/060215_consumer.htm

Substance Abuse and Mental Health Services Administration (SAMHSA). (2009). *Illness management and recovery: How to use the evidence-based practice KITS.* HHS Pub. No. SMA-09–4462, Rockville, MD: Center for Mental Health Services, U.S. Department of Health and Human Services.

Sullivan, H. S. (1947). Therapeutic investigations in schizophrenia. *Journal for the Study of Interpersonal Processes, 10,* 121–125.

Sullivan, P. F., Neale, M. C., & Kendler, K. S. (2000). Genetic epidemiology of major depression: Review and meta-analysis. *American Journal of Psychiatry, 157*(10), 1552–1562.

Sullivan, W. P. (1993). "It helps me to be a whole person": The role of spirituality among the mentally challenged. *Psychosocial Rehabilitation Journal, 16,* 125–134.

Surber, R. W. (Ed.). (1994). *Clinical case management: A guide to comprehensive treatment of serious mental illness.* Thousand Oaks, CA: Sage.

Swann, A. C. (2006). Neurobiology of bipolar depression. In R. S. El-Mallach & N. S. Ghaemi (Eds.), *Bipolar depression: A comprehensive guide* (pp. 37–68). Washington, DC: American Psychiatric Publishing.

Szentagotai, A., & David, D. (2010). The efficacy of cognitive-behavioral therapy in bipolar disorder: A quantitative meta-analysis. *Journal of Clinical Psychiatry, 71*(1), 66–73.

Tager-Flusberg, H., Joseph, R., & Folstein, S. (2001). Current directions on research on autism. *Mental Retardation and Developmental Disabilities Research, 7*(1), 21–29.

Taylor, D. (1997). The psychoanalytic approach to psychotic aspects of the personality: Its relevance to psychotherapy in the National Health Service. In C. Mace & F. Margison (Eds.), *Psychotherapy of psychosis* (pp. 49–62). London: Gaskell.

Thyer, B., & Pignotti, M. (2011). Evidence-based *practices* do not exist. *Clinical Social Work Journal, 39*(4), 328–333.

Torrey, W. C., Rapp, C. A., Van Tosh, L., McNabb, C. R. A., & Ralph, R. O. (2005). Recovery principles and evidence-based practice: Essential ingredients of service improvement. *Community Mental Health Journal, 41*(1), 91–100.

Tyrer, S. (2006). What does history teach us about factors associated with relapse in bipolar affective disorder? *Journal of Psychopharmacology, 20*(Suppl. 2), 4–11.

U.S. Department of Health and Human Services (DHHS). (2001). *Culture, race, and ethnicity: A supplement to mental health: A report of the surgeon general.* http://www.mindfully.org/ Health/Mental-Health-Ethnicity.htm

Uhlhaas, P. J., & Mishara, A. L. (2007). Perceptual anomalies in schizophrenia: Integrating phenomenology and cognitive neuroscience. *Schizophrenia Bulletin, 33*(1), 142–156.

van Os, J., Rutten, B. P., & Poulton, R. (2008). Gene-environmental interactions in schizophrenia: Review of epidemiological findings and future directions. *Schizophrenia Bulletin, 34*(6), 1066–1082.

Vieta, E., & Suppes, T. (2008). Bipolar II disorder: Arguments for and against a distinct diagnostic entity. *Bipolar Disorders, 10,* 163–178.

Virginia Organization of Consumers Advocating Leadership (VOCAL). (2009). *Firewalkers: Madness, beauty, and mystery: Radically rethinking mental illness.* Charlottesville, VA: Author.

Volkmar, F., Chwarska, K., & Klin, A. (2005). Autism in infancy and early childhood. *Annual Review of Psychology, 56,* 315–336.

Wallace, A. C. (1997). *Setting psychological boundaries: A handbook for women.* Westport, CT: Bergin & Garvey.

Wallcraft, J. (1994). Empowering empowerment: Professionals and self-advocacy projects. *Mental Health Nursing, 14,* 6–9.

Walsh, J. (2000). *Clinical case management with persons having mental illness: A relationship-based perspective.* Pacific Grove, CA: Wadsworth-Brooks/Cole.

Walsh, J. (2007). *Endings in clinical practice* (2nd ed.). Chicago: Lyceum Books.

Walsh, J. (2009). Clinical case management. In A. R. Roberts (Ed.), *Social workers' desk reference* (2nd ed.) (pp. 755–759). New York: Oxford.

Wang, J., Iannotti, R., Luk, J. W., & Nansel, T. R. (2010). Co-occurrence of victimization from five subtypes of bullying: Physical, verbal, social exclusion, spreading rumors, and cyber. *Journal of Pediatric Psychology, 35*(10), 1103–1112.

Warner, R. (2009). Recovery from schizophrenia and the recovery model. *Current Opinion in Psychiatry, 22*(4), 374–380.

Wehman, P., Smith, M. D., & Schall, C. (2009). *Autism and the transition to adulthood.* Baltimore: Paul H. Brookes Publishing.

Weiden, P., & Havens, L. L. (1994). Psychotherapeutic management techniques in the treatment of outpatients with schizophrenia. *Hospital & Community Psychiatry, 45*(6), 549–555.

Weissman, M. M., Markowitz, J. C., & Klerman, G. L. (2000). *Comprehensive guide to interpersonal psychotherapy.* New York: Basic Books.

Werbart, A. (1997). Separation, termination process, and long-term outcomes in psychotherapy with severely disturbed patients. *Bulletin of the Menninger Clinic, 61*(1), 16–43.

Werner, C., & Altman, I. (2000). Humans and nature: Insights from a transactional view. In S. Wapner, J. Demick, T. Yamamoto, & H. Minami (Eds.), *Theoretical perspectives in environment-behavior research: Underlying assumptions, research problems, and methodologies* (pp. 21–37). New York: Kluwer Academic.

White, W., Boyle, M., & Loveland, D. (2005). Recovery from addiction and from mental illness: Shared and contrasting lessons. In R. Ralph & P. Corrigan (Eds.), *Recovery in mental illness: Broadening our understanding of wellness.* Washington, DC: American Psychological Association.

Wiggins, J. B., & Cather, S. (2006). Examination of the time between first evaluation and first autistic spectrum disorder diagnosis: A population-based sample. *Journal of Developmental & Behavioral Pediatrics, 27*(2), 79–95.

Wong, D. F. K. (2006). *Clinical case management for people with mental illness: A bio-psycho-social vulnerability stress model.* New York: Haworth Press.

Wong, H. H. L., & Smith, R. G. (2006). Patterns of complementary and alternative medical therapy use in children diagnosed with autism spectrum disorders. *Journal of Autism and Developmental Disorders, 36*(7), 901–909.

Worthington, R. L., Soth, A. M., & Moreno, M. V. (2007). Multicultural counseling competencies research: A 20-year content analysis. *Journal of Counseling Psychology, 54,* 351–361.

Wright-Berryman, J. L., McGuire, A. B., & Salyers, M. P. (2011). A review of consumer-provided services on assertive community treatment and intensive case management teams: Implications for future research and practice. *Journal of the American Psychiatric Nurses Association, 17*(1), 37–44.

Young, A. S., Klap, R., Sherbourne, C. D., & Wells, K. B. (2001). The quality of care for depressive and anxiety disorders in the United States. *Archives of General Psychiatry, 58,* 55–61.

Young, S. L., & Ensing, D. S. (1999). Exploring recovery from the perspective of people with psychiatric disabilities. *Psychiatric Rehabilitation Journal, 22*(3), 219–231.

Youngstrom, E. A., Findling, R. L., Youngstrom, J. K., & Calabrese, J. R. (2005). Toward an evidence-based assessment of pediatric bipolar disorder. *Journal of Clinical Child and Adolescent Psychology, 34*(3), 433–448.

Zimmerman, M. A. (2000). Empowerment theory: Psychological, organizational, and community levels of analysis. In J. Rappaport & E. Seidman (Eds.), *Handbook of community psychology* (pp. 43–65). New York: Kluwer Academic/Plenum.

Zlotnik, J. (2007). Evidence-based practice and social work education: A view from Washington. *Research on Social Work Practice, 17*(5), 625–629.

Index

About the Author

Joseph Walsh is professor of social work at Virginia Commonwealth University in Richmond, teaching courses in direct social work practice and human behavior, among others. Prior to coming to the university Walsh was a full-time clinical social worker for many years, working at several community mental health services and specializing in services to persons with severe mental illness and their families. He continues to focus most of his writing on topics related to his interest area and maintains a small part-time community practice.